Alberto Periccioli

Bye Bye Cellulite

Alberto Periccioli

Bye Bye Cellulite

Understanding what cellulite is to learn how to manage and overcome it with a 360-degree approach

ScienciaScripts

Imprint

Any brand names and product names mentioned in this book are subject to trademark, brand or patent protection and are trademarks or registered trademarks of their respective holders. The use of brand names, product names, common names, trade names, product descriptions etc. even without a particular marking in this work is in no way to be construed to mean that such names may be regarded as unrestricted in respect of trademark and brand protection legislation and could thus be used by anyone.

Cover image: www.ingimage.com

This book is a translation from the original published under ISBN 978-620-0-84089-9.

Publisher:
Sciencia Scripts
is a trademark of
Dodo Books Indian Ocean Ltd. and OmniScriptum S.R.L Publishing group
Str. Armeneasca 28/1, office 1, Chisinau MD-2012, Republic of Moldova, Europe
Printed at: see last page
ISBN: 978-620-5-39237-9

Summary

1. Introduction

a.   Who are they?

Let me introduce myself: I am Alberto Periccioli, I was born in Grosseto in 1976 and I have been working as a Telecommunications Engineer in the IT sector for about twenty years. You are probably a little disoriented and wondering what I have to do with the subject of this book...

In addition to IT, fitness and bodybuilding have fascinated me since I was 16 years old. This is why I studied and deepened these disciplines, obtaining the Personal Trainer and Body Building Instructor certifications, recognised by CONI (Italian National Olympic Committee).

Throughout my life, I have always practised sport and physical activity, taking an interest in everything related to wellbeing: in fact, you cannot perform in your professional life, nor in your private life, if you are not well. If body, mind and soul are in harmony, our relationships with others will also be positively affected and the results we achieve will be far better, as will the quality of our lives.

This is why a holistic approach to the search for wellbeing is necessary: analysing the symptoms of a pathology, for example, is the first step in understanding what is happening, but then we need to establish its causes (aetiology), understand how lifestyle, or some of our attitudes, diet, supplementation, training, the presence of any other pathologies, moods, etc. all contribute to determining a mal-being and how we need to intervene to manage and treat it, where possible.

Well-being must be understood as the best condition attainable by ourselves, in relation to our being and our psycho-physical condition at that particular moment. Each of us represents a *unicum*, and should be respected and treated as such. My well-being will never be the same as yours.

My studies and my approach are directed towards the search for well-being within the society in which we live: we are social animals, we have affections and interests in the context in which we live and we do not necessarily have to become monks or hermit thinkers to be well. We never stop learning, the only certainty is to always put our beliefs and knowledge to the test. Only results obtained through field testing, measured as scientifically and objectively as possible, act as impartial judges, passing judgement without appeal.

What is proposed in this work is the fruit of my research in the *magnum sea of* information (and disinformation), suitably revised and simplified to be accessible to all, after having put it to the test over the years.

b.   Why this book?

There are already many books on this subject: why write another one?

Many of the books that are on the market, even at a very high cost, are in my opinion only written to sell a training method, supplements, a certain diet, or the book itself. Often, the diets, therapies or cures of this or that luminary on duty are proposed, without taking into account the complexity of the pathology called cellulite. In fact, as we will explore in this book, the causes that lead to its formation are multiple; consequently, the approach to treating and curing cellulite must also be multidisciplinary.

Moreover, in many of these works, language is used that is a little too technical and difficult to understand. Often the specialist parades medical terms for his own ego, 'showing off his culture', not creating the conditions for understanding, nor even the basis for a dialogue with the patient, merely displaying an empty eloquence. Rarely are concrete examples given that can be applied in everyday life, except for the most trivial, and hardly any easy-to-use summary diagrams.

These motivations prompted me to write this book, in addition to the fact that I find it my duty to make the knowledge I have learnt over the years available to everyone. Academic studies have been fundamental in training me to obtain the necessary tools to discern and understand what I have studied in the texts of doctors and professionals in the field. For this reason, in each section, I have included references to the main sources of information from which I have drawn, starting with the official position of the ISS (Istituto Superiore di Sanità).

Theory without practice is like talking about love without ever having been in love: it cannot be done by 'hearsay'. That is why the text is not a banal repetition of what has been studied, but an ex-post reworking on a scientific and practical basis.

In this book, I provide my current knowledge on a subject that afflicts about 90% of women: such an impactful problem needs a work that deals with it and addresses it in a scientific way, but one that is easily accessible to all, a bit like in the wonderful episodes of Superquark, the wonderful programme that was once hosted by Piero Angela.

The work is structured with a 'very practical' outlook, i.e. with concrete examples of how to act to counter this annoying blemish, before it becomes a pathology, or how to manage it, by attacking the problem at 360°: diet, supplementation, lifestyle, training, aesthetic treatments, more or less invasive.

Mens sana in corpore sano is the infamous Latin motto we all know. I would add that our soul must also be healthy. We are a very complex whole, a sort of condominium shared by three apartment blocks that must dialogue and get along with each other. Easier said than done, but it is the main objective of our existence and that of those next to us: we are social animals and, as such, day after day we must learn to know, love, respect and help each other, in a coexistence that is as peaceful as possible and harbours good opportunities.

c.   Who is it addressed to?

This book is aimed at all women, but more generally, at anyone who wants to understand what cellulite is, how to deal with it in order to defeat it, or to manage it better. The language used is deliberately simple, although some technical terms are sometimes used, explained in the text and accompanying images. For this reason, it is a work intended for everyone, as it does not go into the specifics of chemical formulas or biological processes, which require special prior knowledge.

The book is structured in several consequential sections, so that one can first acquire the necessary knowledge to understand what cellulite is and what causes it, and finally how to deal with it in order to limit it, or manage it better.

If you already have some theoretical knowledge on the subject, you can jump straight to the sections of interest to you, such as nutrition, supplementation, training, lifestyle and anti-cellulite treatments, where you will find concrete examples that do not require any special previous knowledge.

e.	Important recommendations

This work is the fruit of what I have learnt in these years of study and in-depth study in the field, and therefore has a purely informative purpose: it cannot and will not replace in any way what official medicine proposes. General practitioners, aestheticians, specialists, as well as nutritionists and dieticians, are the only figures one can and must turn to when it comes to nutrition, supplementation and the treatment of any pathologies.

<u>The author therefore disclaims all liability for any use of this work other than as set out in this section.</u>

2. What is cellulite

First of all, the word 'cellulite' is derived from the word 'cell' and the suffix 'ite', which in medical terms indicates inflammation (e.g. tendonitis, arthritis, gastritis, etc.). Thus, the word itself would lead one to think of an inflammation of cells. In reality, this is not quite the case: the situation is a bit more complex, because it depends on the stage of progress.

Figure 1: Cellulite

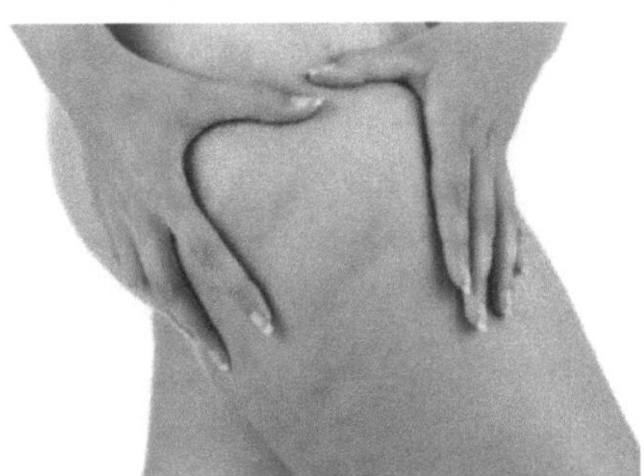

We start with the official position of the Istituto Superiore di Sanità (ISS):

https://www.issalute.it/index.php/la-salute-dalla-a-alla-z-menu/c/cellulite#link-approfondimento

I quote in inverted commas what was published on the above-mentioned page.

<<The condition commonly called cellulite is a skin manifestation localised mainly on the pelvic and abdominal area, hips, buttocks, thighs. It generally presents with micro depressions of the skin, sometimes associated with small nodules of subcutaneous fatty tissue. Due to its visual appearance, it is often referred to as 'orange peel skin', while the scientific name is more properly 'gynoid lipodystrophy', 'oedematous adiposis', 'liposclerosis'.

The variety of designations means that there is still substantial ambiguity as to the causes and true nature of cellulite, it being understood that it is in any case a physiological disorder, typical of women, essentially linked to water retention, accumulation of liquids and micro formations of subcutaneous fat. The term 'cellulite' was introduced in 1922 by Alquier and Paviot, who described it as a simple skin blemish, with no connection to the subcutaneous infection called 'cellulitis' in English medical literature. Numerous clinical examinations in the following decades showed the absence of oedema and fibrosis of any kind.

From a clinical point of view, cellulite manifests itself as a series of uneven areas of the skin, with the presence of subcutaneous micro-cavities arranged perpendicularly to the tissue, as well as very small protuberances of fatty tissue in the skin itself.

In essence, there is no agreement in the medical literature on the correct interpretation of the phenomenon, and to this day cellulite is still a condition that is not fully understood and a decidedly minor topic for medical researchers, so much so that it has very often been called an 'invented disease', or even the 'most investigated non-disease' (Godoy 2012). Scientific publications over the last 30 years highlight that it is a phenomenon with various physiological bases, not a disease, which can be caused, perpetuated or worsened by numerous factors.>>

<u>So, for the ISS, cellulite is not a disease</u>. In fact, it is referred to as an <<invented disease>>.

This is the position of official medicine. But then why do many doctors, even established ones, call it a real <<pathology>>? Who is right?

At the end of this chapter you will find my answer to this question. In the following sections, however, you will find important information to understand in more detail what cellulite is and thus the reasons for my answer.

In this section, in addition to the already mentioned ISS page, I also refer to the following public page of Dr Massimo Spattini, a long-time medical and nutritional luminary who is a true authority on the subject:

https://massimospattini.com/la-cellulite/

Cellulite affects the adipose tissue (fat), which is initially soaked in excess fluid. If not properly treated, the connective tissue can degenerate, becoming dense, fibrous and sclerotic. For this reason, doctors prefer to define cellulite more correctly as *sclerosing fibroedematous panniculopathy*.

If you are not interested in delving into the 'more technical' aspects, you can skip directly to Chapter 3, but I suggest you at least read the following: it will be helpful for a better general understanding of the problem.

a. The 4 basic tissue types

Tissue' is defined as a group of cells that share a similar structure and functions. There are four basic types of tissue in the human body:

- covering or epithelium

- support or connective tissue

- muscular

- nervous

Since cellulite manifests itself visually on the skin, we will treat the epithelium and connective tissue in the following sections, as well as the deeper layer beneath: the adipose tissue.

Do not be frightened if something is not immediately clear: what is set out at the end of paragraph c of this section and what is set out in the following chapters will be understandable anyway.

See the following image:

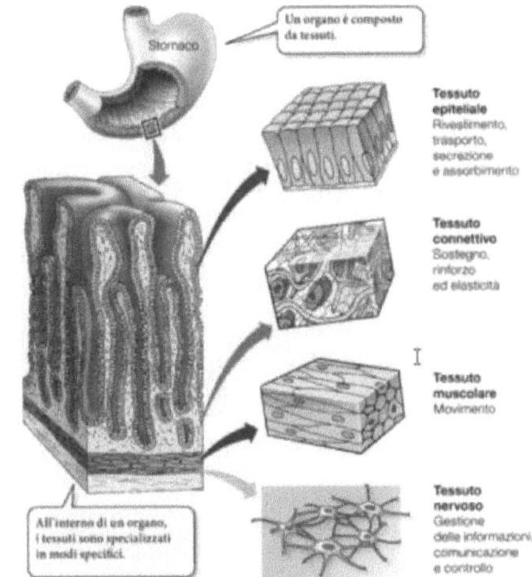

b. The skin

The skin is the envelope that covers our entire body. It consists of three main layers:

- *Epidermis:* is composed of several layers of cells called 'epithelial'. From bottom to top we have the basal, spiny, granular, shiny and horny layer: we will not go into this any further, as it is not necessary for the purposes of the discussion.

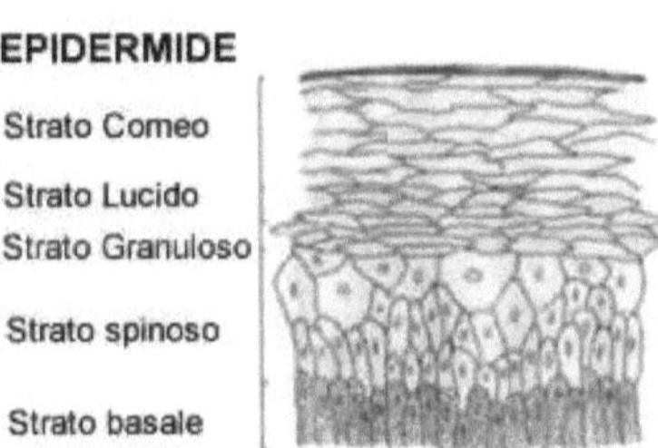

The cells of the epidermis continuously renew themselves, moving up from the basal layer to the surface, taking on the characteristics of the cells in each layer. In healthy skin, the entire cycle lasts about four weeks. The epidermis protects against water loss, UV radiation and the entry of bacteria and fungi.

- *Connective Tissue (or dermis):* is composed of two parts: the *papillary*, located below the epidermis, and the *reticular*, located between the papillary and hypodermis. It contains collagen and elastic fibres, which make it elastic and resistant to traction, as well as firm, thanks to the presence of organic chemical compounds from the sugar family (called *glycosaminoglycans*), which give it hydration and turgidity; it also contains the follicles, glands and hair erector muscles. The dermis transfers nutrients and sebum, an oily substance that protects the surface layer of the skin from bacteria and dehydration, to the epidermis.

o *Hypodermis (or subcutaneous):* is a tissue located below the dermis, consisting of cell clusters, called adipocytes, rich in triglycerides, held together by a scaffold of connective fibres and fluid. The hypodermis is highly vascularised and innervated, performing important functions:

- It is the body's main energy store (in the form of fat -> adipocytes), to be used when needed

- It is a thermal insulator, protecting from the cold (minimising heat loss), or generating heat through the oxidation of triglycerides (chemical reaction that breaks them down using oxygen)

- Provides protection against trauma (e.g. falls or shocks)

- Shaping the body figure

- It affects the body's metabolism

- Makes it possible for the skin to slide on the underlying planes

The drawing in the next figure makes what has just been stated more visually clear:

Figure 4:Cute

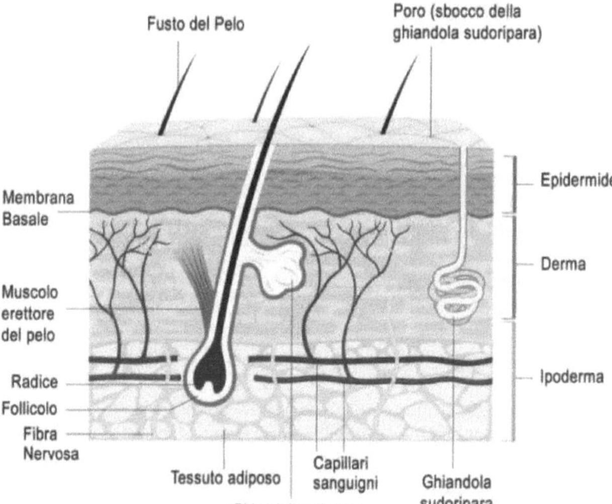

For further information: https://www.my-personaltrainer.it/anatomia/cute.html

c. Adipose tissue

The panniculus adiposus is a layer of adipose connective tissue (i.e. fat) under the skin: it consists of flaps of fat tissue separated by branches of elastic fibres and collagen. The adipose tissue is unevenly distributed. In the presence of cellulite, the fat cells 'swell', press on the microcirculation (the collection of small blood vessels also present in the connective tissue), causing water retention (retention of fluid between the cells) and initial inflammation. Connective tissue is derived from embryonic connective tissue and has functions of connection, support, protection from shocks or falls, nourishment, immune defence, transport of fluids, and energy reserve in case of need.

Please refer to the following two figures for clarity:

Figure 5: Formation of Cellulite

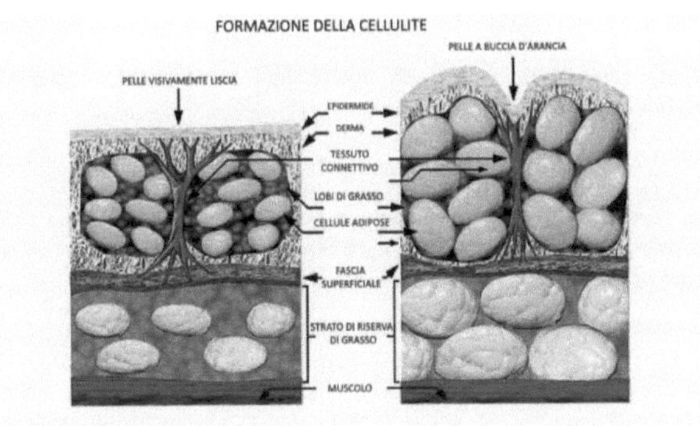

Figure 6: Adipose Tissue (or Panniculus)

In its early stages, cellulite is only a blemish, due to the accumulation of excess fluid between the adipocytes, but as it progresses, it can cause:

- *pain*

- *dermal sclerotization*, i.e. hardening and thickening of the skin; the tissues become fibrous and can no longer slide over each other, so much so that you can no longer pick up a strip of skin between your fingers

- *microcirculation problems*, even major ones

It should now be a little clearer why cellulite should more correctly be called '*sclerosing fibroedematous panniculopathy*': for convenience, we will continue to refer to it as 'cellulite' in the following. Beyond the etymology, which is in any case important, what is important is to understand what it is, the causes, the effects and therefore how to act to limit it, especially in the early stages of its appearance.

It is essential to understand from the outset that when the veins in the legs lose tone, they cause a slowing of blood flow: this also has negative effects on the network of capillaries, which nourishes the panniculus adiposus.

In the presence of loss of venous tone, the small blood vessels tend to dilate, their walls become more porous and permeable, so much so that part of the water escapes from the capillaries and invades the space (called 'interstitial') between the adipocytes (fat cells). The adipose tissue becomes oedematous (full of fluid), losing its normal honeycomb structure: the presence of oedema pulls the adipocytes away from each other and from the capillaries, compressing them (as in figure 4). In this situation, the exchange of nutrients between the adipose tissue and the microcirculation is altered: as the presence of oedema continues, the situation becomes chronic, favouring the stagnation of liquids and waste, which irritate the adipose tissue, to the point of changing its biochemistry and structure.

The connective tissue becomes fibrous, the capillaries become progressively altered, further deteriorating the exchange of oxygen and nutrients with the cells, and eventually clogging up the lymphatic purification system as well. What happens is very similar to what happens when you use a house drain with a clogged sewage system: a disaster! This is why the skin gradually loses elasticity, resulting in the formation of cellulite.

d. Cellulite: real or invented disease?

So, as far as we have seen so far, is cellulite a pathology or not?

As is often the case, in my opinion the truth lies somewhere in between. That is, it depends on the stage of progress of the cellulite itself (a concept that will be analysed in detail in a separate chapter). Initially, in fact, cellulite is just an annoying blemish linked to an excess of interstitial liquids, between the cells of the adipose tissue. As it progresses, however, it can become a real pathology, especially if aggravated by overweight, creating local inflammation and microcirculation problems.

Why does the ISS not consider it a disease?

I think there are essentially two reasons for this: the first is that there is no common agreement among researchers on how to define it, but especially on how to treat it.

Often one is in danger of falling into the hands of people with few scruples, who want to cure something that is not (yet) a real illness, and in order to make money they have no qualms. But this is true in general, even for proven serious illnesses. There is another, perhaps more important reason: the economic one. As we will see in the following chapters, according to reference sources, it is estimated that 80 to 90 per cent of women suffer from cellulite. To date, according to the

https://italiaindati.com/demografia/

There are about 30 million women in Italy, about 5 million of whom are under the age of 19. For the reasons we will see later in the book, doing a rough count, in Italy alone there could be at least 20 million women to be treated: an exorbitant cost for the Italian health service, clearly unsustainable, especially in the absence of a real and definitive cure. There are many doctors, in fact, who consider cellulite a natural process, but not a disease. Moreover, there is currently no drug that can effectively cure it: an exclusively pharmacological therapy would be a useless waste of resources and time.

In support of my thoughts, I report the translation of what was expressed in this important research from 2015:

https://www.ncbi.nlm.nih.gov/pmc/articles/PMC4685482/

<< Cellulite is a complex problem that affects about 85% of women over the age of 20. It occurs mainly on the thighs, buttocks and abdomen and is characterised by an orange peel or cottage cheese appearance.

Cellulite involves multifactorial aetiologies, including genetic predisposition, gender differences, age, ethnicity, diet, sedentary lifestyle and pregnancy. It is characterised by the presence of excess subcutaneous fat swelling in the dermis, blood and lymphatic disorders and altered dermal extracellular matrix.

(…)

It is commonly accepted that the dermal and subcutaneous connective tissue, weakened by an altered and disordered extracellular matrix, plays a key role in the pathophysiology of cellulite and contributes to the uneven and rippled appearance of cellulite-affected skin. Consequently, therapies aimed at restoring the normal structure of the dermis and subcutaneous tissue can be a significant approach to improving the condition of cellulite.

(…)

Although cellulite is often present in healthy, non-obese patients, it is exacerbated by being overweight. Clinical grades of cellulite are positively correlated with body mass index (BMI)

The term cellulite is often used to describe a complex architectural disorder of the skin with multifactorial aetiologies. In general, the formation of cellulite is a natural process and not a disease, which is reflected in an incidence of about 85% in adult females. However, the appearance of cellulite can adversely affect women's quality of life and some suffer severely from their rippled orange peel skin.

The pathophysiology of cellulite is still not entirely clear, but it is generally accepted that, in addition to an altered connective tissue structure and an altered dermal extracellular matrix, being overweight also has a negative effect on cellulite-prone skin areas such as the thighs and buttocks. >>

In this text, unless otherwise indicated, I will consider cellulite as a pathology, i.e. when it is not in its primordial stage of simple blemish.

3. Causes of cellulite

Cellulite has multifactorial causes, so a multidisciplinary approach is needed to combat it.

Among the main causes of the onset or aggravation of cellulite are certainly genetic factors (e.g. hormonal problems), but also lifestyle, postural problems, poor diet, circulation and detoxification problems, prolonged stress, lack of or inadequate training.

Underlying it all, however, is a specific hormonal situation, with oestrogen predominance, as we will analyse in the following sections.

a.   Genetic factors and heredity

Have you ever wondered why women are more prone to cellulite than men?

The cause lies mainly in the greater presence of oestrogen hormones in women's bodies compared to men. These hormones, which are essential for female fertility, promote an accumulation of fat in the hips, up to the knee, triggering potential circulatory problems and promoting water retention.

In young girls, at the age of puberty, the presence of cellulite is almost never detected, whereas in the transition to adolescence it can occur: it corresponds to the increased level of oestrogen hormones. Furthermore, women who are more androgynous (i.e. with not only feminine, but also somewhat 'masculine' characters), with more testosterone and less oestrogen than the average female, do not show cellulite. Similarly, in men with high oestrogen levels, cellulite occurs.

For this reason, heredity plays a fundamental role: the predominance of certain hormones makes a woman take on a particular physical appearance. Think for example of the classic gynoid woman, with a somewhat pear-shaped conformation (no offence intended: this is a definition often given by doctors and nutritionists), i.e. narrower in the upper part of the body, with hips and thighs larger than the shoulders and chest, who tends to accumulate fat with ease, presenting problems of water retention in the legs, swelling and often also oedema accompanied by pain.

Genetics determines our morpho-biotype, i.e. our hormone dosages and consequently our physical structure. Learning how to identify it becomes fundamental, in order to know ourselves, better understand how to behave and what steps to take to manage cellulite (and not only that). For example, a gynoid girl with a mother suffering from cellulite will have a high probability of developing cellulite as she gets older.

b.   Prolonged stress

We have all experienced excessive stress at least once in our lives: who hasn't had an argument with a colleague, friend, acquaintance, husband, wife, children, not to mention those who drive a car without respecting the rules of the road at all?

Stress in itself is not bad; on the contrary, it is our way of adapting to a new situation. However, even if a peak of stress is unhealthy, our body can easily handle it: we come from thousands of years of adaptation, let alone handle the annoyance induced by an undisciplined motorist cutting us off on the road.

Quite different, however, is the case when stress peaks accumulate during the day, becoming a constant background in the daily routine: chronicisation is a serious problem, because it leads to hormonal imbalances, potentially damaging to our health, not only to cellulite.

In fact, following a sudden and unexpected event, such as a honking horn, our organism puts certain hormones into circulation to provide us with an immediate stimulus to action: it is an ancestral heritage, from when we were hunters, but also prey for carnivorous animals. In situations of imminent danger, all energies are made available so that we can react as quickly as possible, as is the case when we need to save ourselves.

In the presence of a sudden event such as the one mentioned above, three hormones are produced by the adrenal glands: cortisol and catecholamines (there are two). Cortisol is produced by the cortical region of the adrenals, on impulse from the brain: the signal starts from the pituitary gland and is propagated by the adrenocorticotropic hormone (ACTH). Catecholamines are produced by the medullary region of the adrenals: these are two hormones (adrenalin and noradrenalin), which together with cortisol prepare the body for exertion.

The combination of these three elements increases heart rate and cardiac output ('the flow rate of pumped blood'), blood pressure, dilation of the bronchi, increasing blood sugar and fats in the blood, as well as glycogen consumption, to improve physical performance and alertness very quickly.

Cortisol has a strong hyperglycaemic power, i.e. it raises blood sugar in the blood stream:

- blood glucose is the concentration of glucose in the blood

- glucose is a monosaccharide, i.e. a sugar that cannot be 'reduced' (technically it is called hydrolysed) into a simpler carbohydrate: it is derived from the reduction of carbohydrates ingested in our bodies, both simple and more complex (such as bread and pasta for example)

- glucose is converted into glycogen (in the liver and cell cytoplasm), a form of sugar that is more easily assimilated by the body

- glycogen is assimilated by our cells to produce energy, including the cells of all our muscles

Glucose therefore represents the privileged form of energy that the body accesses to provide an immediate response to a stress, such as an external one caused by immediate stress, which can become prolonged.

An excess of cortisol, however, produces important undesirable effects in the long run, such as:

- lowering of immune defences

- decreased synthesis (i.e. 'production') of collagen and bone matrix, accelerating osteoporosis

- increases the feeling of tiredness

- increases the concentration of sodium and decreases that of potassium, causing water retention

- promotes protein catabolism (part of the process of protein breakdown and regeneration in the body) by stimulating the conversion of proteins into glucose and thus into glycogen

- stimulates lipogenesis, i.e. the creation of fatty acids and subsequent accumulation of lipids in certain areas of the body, typically the belly in men (in the form of visceral fat, very dangerous for cardiovascular diseases), or the waist, hips and thighs in women

An increase in circulating cortisol also occurs with prolonged fasting, as well as by eating a lot of food in one meal: as mentioned at the beginning of this paragraph, it is not the sporadic event that generates a problem, but its chronicisation.

Diet also plays a role: an excessive intake of animal proteins and high-glycaemic index carbohydrates can increase cortisol concentration.

Limiting sources of stress is therefore healthy from all points of view, also to combat cellulite.

c.   Lifestyle

Lifestyle has a great influence on the formation of cellulite, with sedentariness being one of the main causes.

Poor mobility slows down metabolism, the elimination of excess fluid and waste materials: the body continuously repairs, destroys and recreates cells, as well as the 'bricks' that make them up, i.e. proteins.

Our foot is the terminal of a blood pump, which continues along the calf and joints: with movement, the pump is activated, stimulating the microcirculation, bringing nutrients to the cells, reducing fluid stasis, and thus fighting the formation of cellulite.

Smoking is a great ally of cellulite: in fact, it creates tissue hypoxia, i.e. it creates a lack of oxygen in the body's tissues and, as seen in the previous paragraphs, this promotes the formation of cellulite in the long run.

Alcohol and water retention are related problems: frequent consumption of alcohol and spirits can strain the microcirculation and promote the formation of the hated orange peel.

Underwear that is too tight, such as briefs or thongs that leave marks on the skin, compresses the lymphatic tissues, preventing the proper drainage of toxins. For the same reason, it would be better to avoid bras with straps that are too thin in relation to the weight of the décolleté: by restricting circulation, they encourage cellulite on the arms. Belts or trousers that are too tight, such as jeans or leggings, can also cause fluid stagnation and water retention: it is better to wear loose trousers, skirts or dresses.

Being overweight certainly favours the onset of cellulite: generally, there is both a stagnation of excess fluid and an accumulation of fat, resulting in an increase in the volume of fat cells.

Posture also plays an important role. For example, those who have lumbar hyperlordosis (a very pronounced S-curve formed between the lower back and the buttocks) tend to bring the organs inside the abdominals forward, compressing the veins in the pelvis and thus promoting poor blood circulation, leading to cellulite. There are four types of posture-related situations and attitudes to take into account, because in the long run they can contribute to the appearance of cellulite, or aggravate it if already present:

1- Sitting at the PC for many hours a day: slows down the circulation. Poor posture can encourage the accumulation of fat on the hips and buttocks. Sitting for a couple of hours is no problem, but eight consecutive hours is quite different.

2- Standing still for many hours a day: Equivalent to the previous point from the point of view of circulation and what goes with it.

3- Wearing high heels: they hinder the correct support of the sole of the foot, as well as the correct movement of the calf muscle, which is essential for pushing the blood up from the lower limbs. The ideal would be to wear a heel no higher than 3 or 4 centimetres, not too tight.

4- Keeping your legs crossed: often and for a long time, it hinders blood circulation.

We often hear that drinking a lot helps eliminate excess fluid and water retention.

Just as often, one hears that eliminating salt is a good rule in order not to induce water retention and thus cause or worsen cellulite.

Is this really how things are?

In fact, some salt is absolutely necessary in the diet, just as drinking too much, or too little, can alter the water-salt balance and excess extra-cellular fluid.

We will look again at the causes that lead to cellulite accumulation in the chapter on the lifestyle to adopt in order to combat this pathology, providing specific suggestions.

4. Who suffers from cellulite?

As we have mentioned in previous sections of the book, about 90 per cent of women are affected by cellulite and, of these, almost all after the age of puberty.

Source:

https://www.ansa.it/canale_saluteebenessere/notizie/lei_lui/medicina/2018/05/03/il-90-delle-donne-ha-la-cellulite-guida-per-contrastarla_57ac781a-348d-417e-b539-0e1675e6d1ba.html

According to the ISS, at the URL given at the beginning of this book, the estimate would be slightly lower and would be between 80 and 85 per cent.

And the men?

Only 10% of men would be affected.

The problem is essentially hormonal, linked to oestrogen predominance: individuals with higher oestrogen levels are more easily affected. This is in fact the case for men suffering from gynaecomastia, i.e. enlarged breasts.

In a way, it is the dual case of baldness, from which men suffer more than women, for different but still genetic and hormonal reasons.

Observing bodybuilding stage athletes, muscular, defined and totally devoid of cellulite, one might think to increase the testosterone level in women, but it might not be a good idea: in fact, seeing them shave their beards like men, or speak in an even lower voice than men, might be 'un-feminine'.

Better to let nature take its course, adopting lifestyles and small daily changes from a young age to prevent this disease.

5. Effects of cellulite

Cellulite presents itself with so-called 'orange peel skin' (see figure 7), which can be more or less pronounced. In minor cases, the dimples of the skin are barely visible; in more severe cases, however, they are considerable in size and hard to the touch.

Figure 7: Normal Skin Vs Cellulite

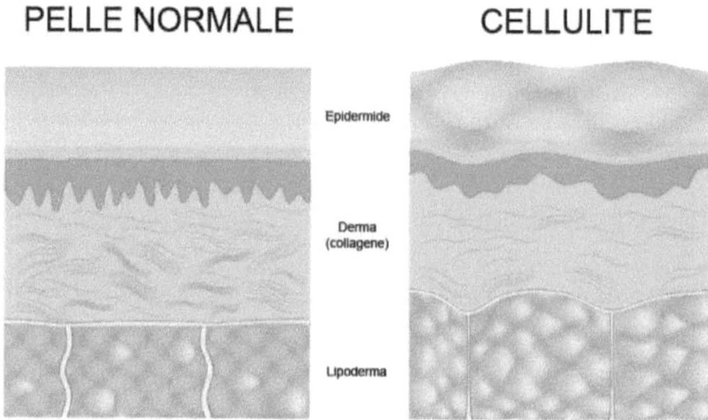

Although cellulite is considered a blemish, it can become a real health problem. The exaggerated growth of the panniculus adiposus, in fact, can compromise the lymphatic and venous circulation, causing oedema and nerve compression, producing pain. Moreover, in the most severe cases and associated with great obesity, it can affect the proper mobility of the legs and joints, such as the knees and hips, causing joint problems in the long run.

The inflammatory state induced at a local level can also have negative effects at a general level: prolonged stagnation of liquids and cellular waste, poor oxygenation and malnutrition of increasingly large areas affected by cellulite can compromise the balance of the entire organism, especially in the severely obese.

There is another effect to consider, which is far from negligible: the psychological one. Many girls and women suffering from cellulite are strongly conditioned by it, so much so that they have problems with self-acceptance and sometimes with their relationships with other people: just think of the limitations they often impose on themselves in terms of clothing, if not even food deprivation or places/events where they have to show off their bodies to others, such as gyms, spas, the sea, etc., negatively affecting the quality of their lives and with important psychological and social implications.

On this subject, I leave the URL of a funny sketch in which Franco Califano together with Daniele Luttazzi rehabilitate and ennoble cellulite:

https://vm.tiktok.com/ZMFkKWsoN/

Even an imperfection can be liked, sometimes more than perfection...

6. Cellulite stages

How to recognise cellulite and its developmental stage?

Let us start once again with the above-mentioned ISS page.

<<There is little to be said about the symptoms of cellulite, since it is not an actual disease but rather a skin blemish. Of course, palpation of the skin, as well as an examination by a dermatologist, can highlight the areas of the body where it occurs most frequently: mainly the buttocks, thighs, abdomen and hips. Normally, cellulite is classified according to a four-level scale created by Nürnberger and Müller in 1978:

0 = no signs of cellulite

1 = the skin is smooth but signs of cellulite appear by pinching the skin or contracting the muscles

2 = cellulite introflections are present and visible even without stressing the skin

3 = presence of the alterations of stage 2 in greater numbers and over a larger area, accompanied by the presence of nodules

According to other classifications, the level of blemishes and skin changes can be measured in density, size, depth, tissue laxity and other physiological parameters.

In the hypothesis that considers cellulite an oedematous-fibro-sclerotic panniculopathy, the evolution and/or degeneration of the phenomenon is classified as follows:

oedematous, cellulite is only noticeable to the touch, at this stage, fluid stagnation in the tissues prevails with localised swelling and oedema, especially around the ankles, calves, thighs and arms

fibrous, due to liquids penetrating the tissues, the cells become distanced from each other and can no longer perform their metabolic functions. The elastic fibres that make the skin soft and taut are compressed by the fat cells; the collagen fibres, which perform a supporting function, degenerate and the capillaries are altered; small nodules form, which are not perceptible to the touch except as subcutaneous roughness, and so-called orange peel skin

sclerotic, where it forms a sclerosis the tissue becomes hard to the touch with the appearance of large nodules; the skin surface takes on the typical 'mattress-like' appearance with hollows and patches of colour, is cold and painful to the touch >>

From my point of view, this turns out to be a good explanation, but not an easy one to use for an initial self-analysis. That is why I provide below a restatement and summary of the two theories above, with a final easy-to-follow summary outline, which can be printed out and used for appropriate self-assessment if necessary.

So let us now treat the 4 stages of cellulite:

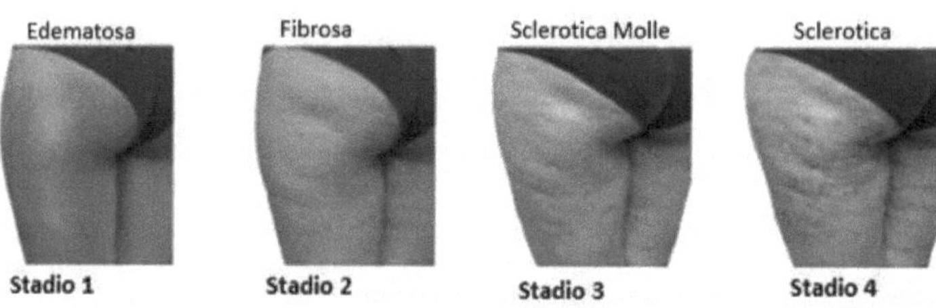

a.   Stage 0

This phase indicates the absence of cellulite. The blood flows unimpeded in the capillaries, passing through the adipose tissue and allowing proper metabolic exchanges between the cells. This stage is therefore not considered for cellulite.

b.   Stage 1 or oedematous cellulite

This is the initial phase in which fluid stagnation in the tissues prevails. Cellulite can only be felt by touch; localised swellings (oedemas) can be seen, mainly around the ankles, calves, thighs and arms. In a standing person, cellulite is not noticeable, but if you plica the skin (i.e. pinch the skin) you can detect the 'orange peel' appearance. The walls of the blood vessels become more permeable, allowing the fluid in the blood vessels to penetrate the surrounding tissues, causing a thickening of the tissue due to the accumulation and stagnation of plasma in the interstitial spaces (i.e. between the cells).

Adipocytes accumulate lipids (triglycerides) inside them, increasing in volume and quantity. In fact, excess fat swells the adipose cells up to 50 times their original size, altering circulation and causing toxins to accumulate, resulting in local inflammation. This situation can occur when caloric intake is higher than energy consumption, over a prolonged period of time.

Signs: the skin is more doughy and cold to the touch; compressing or stiffening the muscle, the characteristic 'orange peel' signs appear. If the skin is plumped, it is soft and painless, but there is less elasticity. Pressing with the fingertip on the skin leaves the impression of a dimple for a longer time, especially on the inner thigh. Dimples, stretch marks, pale, dry or oily skin can then be seen.

Symptoms: they are not visible at this stage.

Reversible? This phase is curable and completely reversible.

c.   Stage 2 or fibrous cellulitis

This is the phase in which the characteristic 'orange peel' appearance of the skin becomes clearly visible, without the need to peel it.

Excess fluid accumulated within the tissues in stage 1 leads to swelling of the tissues and the area affected by cellulite swells (e.g. swollen legs). The excess fluid pushes the adipocytes away, resulting in depressions on the surface, which are more pronounced the larger the fat cells are. Refer to figure 5 and imagine adipocytes as potatoes growing underground. If the soil in which they are located is swollen with liquid, the potatoes move and the soil on the surface is affected, resulting in depressions. If the size of the potatoes increases, the depressions become even more pronounced: this is how orange peel is created.

The size of the adipocytes increases essentially for two reasons: the first is an excessive intake of calories compared to the required consumption, over a prolonged period of time; the second is linked to the first, because a vicious circle is triggered, in which the adipocytes, as they swell, compress the capillaries, worsening the venous circulation. The capillaries will ooze plasma, which will spill along with toxins into the interstitial spaces (the spaces between the cells), further 'clogging' the local lymphatic and venous system, which is already compromised under these conditions. In this situation, the fats accumulated in the cells are used with difficulty by the organism for energy purposes, and will inevitably tend to accumulate, leading to further deterioration, thus establishing a dangerous vicious circle.

I reproduce figure 5 again for convenience:

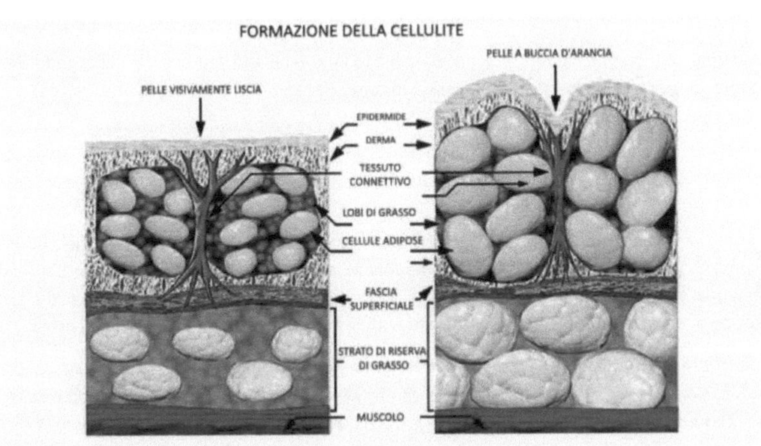

It is clear from the figure that the enlargement and removal of fat cells leads to the formation of so-called orange peel skin.

In this phase, the skin can take on a pale, cold and doughy appearance; it becomes poorly elastic, small subcutaneous nodules form (not perceptible to the touch, except as roughness), a sign of poor blood circulation and water retention that swells the fat cells. Water retention leads to an accumulation of waste and inflammation of the tissues. This cellulite is still not very noticeable and is mainly located on the belly, arms, thighs, hips and buttocks.

Signs: the skin shows the characteristic signs of 'orange peel', with more or less evident depressions. The skin is not uniform in colour and may show slight changes in skin tone (called dyschromia).

Symptoms: squeezing the areas affected by cellulite may induce some pain. The skin in these areas is cooler to the touch than in the surrounding areas and discolourations may occur.

Reversible? This phase is curable and reversible, provided action is taken in good time.

d.   Stage 3 or soft sclerotic cellulite

At this stage, the nodules become larger, about the size of grains of rice, and hardened, causing pain to the touch. Signs of venous and/or lymphatic insufficiency may appear, with oedema of the tissues. The venous tone may then be insufficient.

Signs: the part affected by cellulite is soft, lacking in tone; many nodules and hollows are present; the 'orange peel' is very evident, even without compression. Bruising may appear: if present, this indicates circulatory insufficiency.

Symptoms: pain to the touch, cold and discoloured skin (dyschromia). Excess fluid is very evident around the cellulite clusters.

Reversible? Although with difficulty, it is possible to intervene and improve the initial condition. In some cases it can be cured and regressed, in others it can only be managed and limited.

e.   Stage 4 or sclerotic cellulitis

In this phase there is an aggravation of the signs indicated in the previous one. The nodules become macro-nodules, increasing considerably in size (comparable to a pea) and spread. Pressing at the nerve endings increases the pain to the touch. Dimples appear, so that the skin takes on a 'mattress' appearance: in fact, the nodules reproduce and unite with each other.

Signs: these are the same as in stage 3, but more marked and diffuse, to the extent that the skin tends to take on a so-called 'mattress' appearance, with a purplish colour; if it is pinched it causes pain. There is no longer a marked excess of extracellular fluid, as in the previous stages.

Symptoms: the same as stage 3, but pressing at the nerve endings increases the pain to the touch. Cellulitis is typically located on the thighs, buttocks and inner part of the knee; the skin is purplish in the affected areas. Palpating and pinching the skin, it is easy to feel knots the size of a pea.

Reversible? No! Unfortunately, this phase is too advanced to be reversible, unless surgical or similar treatments are carried out, which we will see in the later sections of the book: one can only mitigate the effects, particularly the pain.

A practical summary is given in *Table 1:*

Table 1: Stages of cellulite

Cellulite stage	Signs	Symptoms	Reversible
1) Edematous	Pale, doughy, cold skin to the touch; orange peel only by compressing the area or tightening the muscle	Not present	YES, completely
2) Fibrous	Pale, pasty and cold skin to the touch; orange peel also present on the feet; slight discolouring	Pain to the touch; areas with cellulite colder than surrounding areas	YES, if caught in time
3) Soft Sclerotic	Area with softer cellulite than the other areas; many lumps and hollows; very noticeable orange peel. Excess fluid evident around the cellulite clusters. Noticeable nodules similar in size to grains of rice.	Cold skin; dyschromia; pain to the touch	YES, partially
4) Sclerotic	Aggravation of stage 3 signs; mattress-like skin. Irregular, orange-peel surface. Dimples, stretch marks, pale, dry or oily skin. Nodules also evident to the touch, comparable in size to a pea.	Aggravation of symptoms stage 3; severe pain at nerve endings. Purple skin in affected areas.	NO (except for surgery or similar, which we will see in the last part of the book)

7. Preventing and treating cellulite

We have now reached the long-awaited chapter, the focus of the book: is it possible to prevent cellulite? And if it has already appeared, can it be cured?

An answer, albeit partial, has already been given in the previous chapter: it is important to intervene early, when the first signs appear. Once cellulite has gained too much of a foothold, it unfortunately becomes difficult, if not impossible, to get it to recede without surgery or similar.

Good lifestyle practices should be adopted from an early age in order to avoid, or at least delay, the onset of the actual disease.

How to do it? The approach must be holistic, to deal with the problem at 360°, through:

- Power supply
- Integration
- Physical Exercise
- Lifestyle
- Aesthetic and Therapeutic Treatments

Tackling the problem in the hope of solving it by adopting only a good diet, or only adequate physical training, or only quality aesthetic treatments, will inexorably lead to failure and frustration: we will spend energy and money in vain. Undoubtedly, we will experience an improvement, we will benefit in terms of aesthetics and general health, but unless we intervene in stage I or stage II (as long as it is not already too advanced), we will be disappointed.

Therefore, the first step is to have oneself assessed by an expert in the field, possibly an aesthetic doctor, in a qualified centre. This step is essential, because unless one has some experience in this regard, the self-assessment may not be objective and some pathologies related to this disease may remain hidden. Think of possible circulation problems, with poor venous tone, or the presence of possible oedemas causing pain: these are all signs that should not be underestimated, understood and treated appropriately, but also promptly.

We learn to treat cellulite for what it is, when it manifests itself: a real disease, fortunately often curable, or one with which it is possible to live, without it worsening.

In the next sections of this chapter, we will take a detailed look at how to attack cellulite in every respect, through hints and tips that can be put into practice in daily life.

a.   Power supply

Nutrition plays a key role in counteracting the appearance of cellulite, as well as in treating it wherever possible.

It must be made clear from the outset, however, that there are no pre-constituted diets that are suitable for all people, or that are magical and have an immediate effect. As we have analysed in the previous chapters, the problem is linked to several factors, including not only diet, but also hormonal processes and lifestyle, which are intrinsically linked. Moreover, the more deep-rooted the cellulite is, the more it is necessary to change habits and behaviour: only the constant application of rules, aimed at healthy living, leads to tangible and lasting effects.

Consistent treatment, well-dosed exercise and proper nutrition gradually change the tissues, maintaining the results obtained.

If cellulite is present in an individual who is neither overweight nor severely overweight, it is inadvisable to undertake low-calorie diets. It is more important, in fact, to have quality food, without overdoing the quantity.

For further information: https://massimospattini.com/grasso-e-cellulite/

Once again, it is always good to repeat, it is essential to turn to the only professionals who can help us: nutritionists and dieticians. Below, I will list a number of suggestions for good nutrition to combat cellulite, taken from the books I have read on the subject and from the following and already mentioned source: https://massimospattini.com/cellulite-i-10-comandamenti/

i. Which foods are preferred?

The following general indications have been gathered from training courses in which I have participated, or from advice from doctors and nutritionists in trade magazines, TV, social media, books, etc.

It is good to favour foods rich in fibre, such as fruit, vegetables and whole-grain cereals. Compatible with your physical activity, calorie regime, and the presence of any illnesses, allergies and intolerances, it might be a good idea to eat:

— at least two fruits in the day, preferably, but not necessarily, in the morning and away from main meals

— a good ration of vegetables, one raw and one cooked, at the two main meals of the day

— wholegrain carbohydrates, such as pasta, rice, but also buckwheat, barley, millet, spelt, oats, at lunch more than at dinner: this is a general rule, which may have appropriate exceptions depending on the person's morpho-biotype and state of health; within the week, wholegrain cereals may be replaced once or twice by more refined cereals, provided they are appropriately combined with other foods

— at least once a day protein: preferably at dinner, giving preference in this order to lean fish (anchovies, sole, cod, sea bass, etc.), white meat (chicken, turkey, rabbit), soya, low-fat cheese (low-fat cottage cheese, cottage cheese) and eggs (soft-boiled or boiled)

The above indications are certainly good suggestions for a person who mainly leads a sedentary life. In the case where the individual trains in the morning, introducing a good amount of carbohydrates and protein immediately after training may be a good idea. In the case of training in the evening, just before dinner, it is a good idea to replenish the carbohydrates and not just the protein in the evening meal. Obviously, everything also depends on the type of training, but as a general guideline, it is suggested to take an adequate amount of carbohydrates (minimally also simple ones, such as honey or fruit juices) immediately after training. Carbohydrates, proteins and fats should, in fact, be present at every meal, in the right percentage, i.e. the one appropriate to one's current condition, morphological structure and hormonal constitution. If we know how to do this and know ourselves well, then we are autonomous in preparing our food plan, otherwise, if we do not even know where to start, it is a good idea to turn to professionals in the field, such as nutritionists. In the case of resistance training, the protein quota could increase in relation to age and be spread out over the day.

For more information:

https://pubmed.ncbi.nlm.nih.gov/32666115/

https://pubmed.ncbi.nlm.nih.gov/26797090/

https://pubmed.ncbi.nlm.nih.gov/24015719/

We always use common sense: these 'rules' should not be experienced as restrictions or impositions. They are guidelines, quite general, to try to stay healthy, feel good and full of energy, with the will to face the day and not to suffer it passively: if we eat well, our organism and our mood will be better, as will our relationships with other people; our self-esteem will also be better and we will be more gratified, thus entering a virtuous circle.

If, on the other hand, we continuously feed our organism with junk food, we enter a vicious circle: the worse we eat, the more we are tempted to continue, debilitating our physique, worsening our psycho-physical condition and, ultimately, losing self-esteem and self-confidence, to the point of no longer liking ourselves and having difficulties in social relationships, becoming depressed and unmotivated, and even developing potentially very serious illnesses.

This is why it is good to live our change with serenity and confidence: embracing a new, healthier lifestyle means taking care of ourselves, loving ourselves and respecting ourselves. Once we are in optimal physical condition, we can introduce in moderation certain foods that were 'banned' during the initial change phase, so that we can vary our diet as much as possible and gratify ourselves, without detracting from our pleasure.

ii. The 80/20 rule

A simple and easy to put into practice rule for the judicious introduction of 'banned' foods into the diet is the 80/20 rule, i.e. 80% of the time I introduce good, nutritionally high quality foods into my body, while the remaining 20% I introduce the other foods, which in any case give me pleasure and allow me a harmonious, joyful and not sad social life.

An example is shown in the figure below:

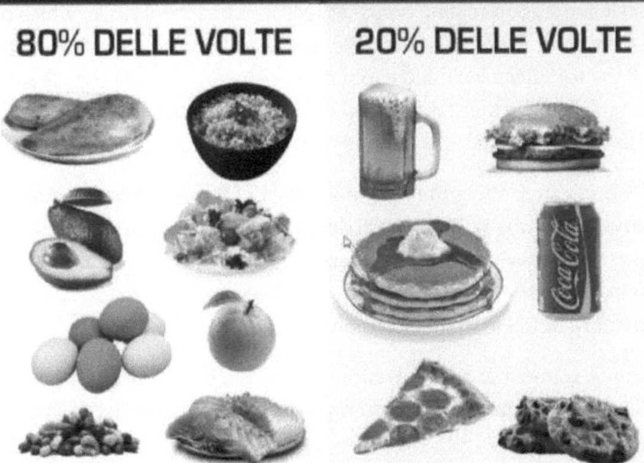

Let us now see how to put this simple rule into practice during the week.

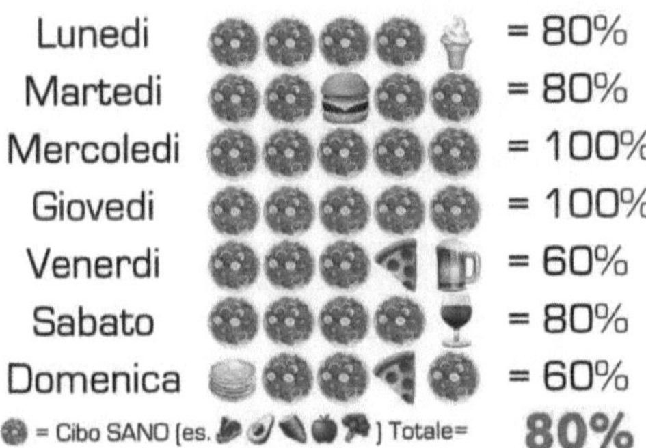

As we can see from the figure above, the goal is to eat healthily for an average of 80% within the week. We can therefore construct a model week, in which some days we try to be 100%, others perhaps 80%, and still others 60%: the important thing is that the weekly average is around 80%.

Once again, what must guide us is common sense. If one day I decide to go out with friends and I am unable to eat and drink as I would like (I deliberately do not use the verb 'duty', because it should not be experienced as an obligation, but rather as a conscious choice), perhaps I can introduce less noble foods and drinks into my body: let us accept this day with joy and pleasure, let us live it and enjoy it. In fact, one day will not destroy the constant work of months or years, on the contrary, it will fortify it, because we will realise that our body, once in shape, is able to tolerate even an 'unhealthy' day well. This will give us satisfaction and new awareness, it will be very gratifying and leave a good feeling on us, as well as a beautiful smile, which others will also notice. Initially, some of us may experience the so-called 'indulgence' with a sense of guilt: let us learn not to call the tolerance included in our diet negative, because even the less noble foods are important, especially on a mental and social level, two fundamental factors for our health and well-being.

Let us learn to keep negative thoughts and feelings of guilt away from us: they will inevitably surface, let us acknowledge them, note them down if it makes us feel better, but then let them flow and go away peacefully. Just as they appeared, they will disappear: let us not pass judgement on them, let us try to observe them as if we were external spectators. We will deal with this aspect in more detail in the chapter on lifestyle.

To summarise: after a somewhat tougher initial phase, once we reach the regime, i.e. the best possible state of fitness for us at the time, managing food within our diet will become easier and more satisfying.

Important note: this rule originated as an extension of the so-called 'Pareto principle', an empirical statistical formula that originated in the socio/economic sphere thanks to Vilfredo Pareto (an Italian economist, sociologist and engineer who lived in the late 1800s and early 1900s) and was extended to various other areas, including the food industry. In training courses in which I have taken part, it has been explained to me by nutritionists in the fitness industry and, finding it very useful, I quote it for the benefit of all.

iii. How to cook food?

Simple cooking would be best: steaming is certainly the best, but cooking in foil, in the oven or in non-stick pans is also fine. Do not use oil in cooking if possible, better if used raw; use olive oil (EVO) for cooking, but avoid smoking it, as it could become unsafe for your health: it is always better to use raw EVO oil on food.

iv. How many meals a day?

Smaller meals are better than 2 or 3 large meals: this limits cortisol peaks, stimulates the metabolism and does not strain the digestive system. So it is better to opt for 5 or 6 meals a day.

Once again, this is a general rule: there are people who are perfectly happy with three meals a day and who, for reasons of time, cannot do otherwise. We must always be able to adapt and make the best of every situation.

v. How much water to drink?

We start again with the official position, which can be found at the following URL:

https://www.salute.gov.it/portale/temi/p2_6.jsp?lingua=italiano&id=4460&area=acque_pota bili&menu=dieta

<< The reference values, which consider total water intake - either through direct consumption or through food and drink of all kinds - under conditions of moderate environmental temperatures and average levels of physical activity, are defined as follows:

- infants up to six months of age: 100 mL/kg per day,
- children:
- between 6 months and one year of age: 800-1000 mL/day,
- between 1 and 3 years of age: 1100-1300 mL/day,
- between 4 and 8 years of age: 1600 mL/day;
- ages 9-13 years: 2100 mL/day for children and 1900 mL/day for girls
- girls;
- adolescents, adults and the elderly:
- females 2 L/day
- males 2.5 L/day.

These values are indicative; in hot climates and intense physical activity, or other conditions that induce dehydration, the levels of water intake may vary considerably (it may be more than double the indicated values). This is also the case under conditions of stress and gastro-enteric disturbances leading to vomiting and diarrhoea, such as infant diarrhoea.>>

Some of the following information was freely taken from 'WATER AS A FOOD by Rosa Inguaggiato and Gioacchino Leandro of the Clinical Nutrition Outpatient Clinic, Body Weight Management and Lifestyle Modification at UOC of Gastroenterology 1 - IRCCS De Bellis - Castellana Grotte', available at this URL:

https://webaigo.it/download/20180806164853.pdf

We often hear that drinking a lot of water is good for you and that you should drink at least two litres a day, preferably more. As far as cellulite is concerned, drinking too much, or too little, leads to a negative result in both cases. It is necessary to hydrate properly: the human body is mainly composed of water (approx. 60% adult males, approx. 50-55% females, approx. 75% infants).

A simple calculation can be applied for self-adjustment:

1 litre of water for every 1,000 Kcal consumed

Therefore, an individual consuming 1,500Kcal/day will have to drink 1.5 litres of water (die = day).

If you do not know your daily calorie intake (but it would be good to know), then you can use this formula, which is based on body weight (it is the one I find most convenient and easy to use):

Body weight in kg x 0.03 = Litres of water needed daily

Thus, an individual weighing 55 kg should consume about 1.65 litres of water per day.

This formula is widely used in the fitness world for simple reference. You can also find a reference to this formula here:

https://www.bereacqua.org/fabbisogno-idrico-giornaliero-formula/

When counting our fluid intake and intake, the food we eat, but also the physical activity we perform or the environmental situation in which we find ourselves must also be taken into account. For example, 500-700 ml and 800-1,500 ml respectively can be obtained from food and drink, to which approximately 350 ml/day of endogenous water must be added.

Endogenous water is derived from the oxidation of nutrients and is produced, in varying proportions, for each gram of metabolised macronutrient:

- 1 ml water for lipids
- 0.55 ml for carbohydrates
- 0.41 ml for protein

Carrying out this calculation becomes extremely complex, unless one has an accurate diet plan, which is why a rough estimate of the endogenous water produced is used.

In addition, water consumption increases if physical activity takes place. Physical activity generates heat: in order to prevent an excessive rise in body temperature, the body increases sweating; sweat evaporates, taking heat away from the body. The evaporation of one gram of sweat from the surface of the skin subtracts approximately 0.6 calories from the body. In this case, during training it is good to listen to yourself and drink as much as your body requires.

Another case to consider is when one is at high altitude: at an altitude above 2,500 metres, both the excretion of urine and the frequency of breathing increase, with a consequent increase in water loss from the body. In fact, exhaled water vapour contains water, which is eliminated through this channel in the range of 250 ml - 350 ml per day.

The need for water also increases on all occasions when there is an increase in sweating, in addition to physical activity, such as during febrile states or particularly hot climates.

Also in the case of diarrhoea or vomiting, there is an increased loss of fluid, which has to be replenished.

Not all people have a good sensibility to meet their body's demand for water; therefore, some resort to the stratagem of drinking a glass of water every two waking hours (about 0.2 litres per glass).

Is there a maximum limit of water to drink daily?

Yes, and is estimated using the following formula:

Body weight in kg x 0.05 = Maximum litres of water that can be drunk daily

Our 55 kg individual should not drink more than 2.75 litres of water per day.

<u>Schematically</u>:

Peso corporeo in kg x 0,03 = Min Litri di Acqua al Giorno [quantità minima]

Peso corporeo in kg x 0,05 = Max Litri di Acqua al Giorno [quantità massima]

vi. Which water to drink?

Preferably mineral, non-carbonated, at room temperature. It can also be taken, in part, in the form of an infusion: green tea, cherry stalks, birch, dandelion, burdock, fennel, ginkgo biloba, rose hips, karkadè, etc.

vii. When to drink?

In scientific circles, it is sometimes recommended to drink away from meals so as not to dilute the gastric juices too much and thus slow down digestion: water intake, at least at main meals, will be provided mainly by fruit and vegetables.

Learning to listen to our bodies and learning to drink as needed becomes essential, without focusing too much on when - also to avoid unnecessary excess anxiety and stress - but rather on the feeling of thirst or dry mouth. Nevertheless, it is good practice to drink:

— As soon as you wake up

— Before the meal

— Before, during and after physical activity

— Between meals

I think these 'recommendations' are quite obvious...

viii. Which foods and drinks should be restricted?

It should be abolished or limited as much as possible:

— alcohol

— fritters

— coffee

— cream

— charcuterie

- chocolate

- confectionery (all)

- mayonnaise

- packaged sauces

- cooking nuts

- canned foods

- subs

- preserves

Seen like this, it looks like a list of prescriptions, forcing us to live a miserable life... As always, common sense must be used: unless there are other serious illnesses, introducing these foods or drinks sparingly over the course of a week is entirely possible, as analysed in 'The 80/20 rule'. Consuming one fried food a week, or one or two coffees a day, may even be good for you. Therefore, one must take these indications *cum grano salis*, as the ancient Romans taught.

ix. Should salt be avoided completely?

Absolutely not!

According to the WHO (World Health Organisation), we should consume no more than 5 grams of table salt, or the equivalent of one teaspoon, every day.

<< The World Health Organisation (WHO) recommends consuming **less than 5 grams of salt per day**, between that already present in food and that added, as much as one teaspoon, corresponding to about **2 grams of sodium per day.**>>

Source:
https://www.salute.gov.it/portale/temi/p2_6.jsp?id=5520&area=stiliVita&menu=alimentazion e

5 grams of table salt corresponds to approximately 2 grams of sodium.

The fact is that salt is contained in almost all food products we consume, especially in packaged products from the food industry. This is why many nutritionists, doctors and experts suggest eating without added salt.

However, a minimum amount of sodium is indispensable for the proper functioning of our cells. In fact, the cell membranes contain the so-called '**sodium-potassium** pump', i.e. a chemical-physical pump that continuously pushes sodium ions out of the cell and potassium ions into the cell. This is why the right balance between sodium and potassium is so important: an imbalance in favour of sodium, with a build-up of sodium ions in the extracellular matrix, can in the long run lead to water retention and cause cellulite.

Another important aspect to consider is that the sodium-potassium pump is driven by '**ATP**' (adenosine triphosphate). Without going into too much detail, the ATP molecule is the most important source of energy in our cells, to the extent that our body synthesises ATP all the time, at all times of the day, even now that you are reading this book. ATP is produced through what is known as '**cellular respiration**', a combustion process resulting from the digestion of food ingested during meals, which leads to the breakdown of food into elementary components, such as simple sugars, amino acids and fatty acids: these are broken down into even simpler molecules, resulting in energy available to the cells in the form of ATP.

For every ATP molecule that is broken down, the pump moves three sodium ions out of the cell and two potassium ions into the cell. When the sodium level drops in the cell, an electrical gradient and a concentration gradient are created: both are used for different purposes, for example for the production of nerve signals. Axons are extensions of neurons, analogous to conducting cables. Nerve axons excrete sodium ions to allow them to re-enter during the nerve impulse, through special channels, the opening of which is controlled by a voltage. The sodium-potassium pump is responsible for keeping the axon ready to transmit the next signal. The gradient helps control the osmotic pressure[1] within the cells and activates a variety of other pumps, which link the flow of sodium to the transport of different molecules, such as calcium ions or glucose.

[1] osmotic pressure can be seen as the 'force' required to prevent liquid from crossing the cell membrane, which is semi-permeable

In conclusion, it is crucial not to exceed the amounts of sodium, but also not to exceed the amounts of potassium, which could even cause very serious heart problems.

In order not to overdo it with salt, we can use fresh raw herbs to season dishes: basil, parsley, rosemary, thyme, oregano, etc.

Attention must be paid to the 'hidden salt' in packaged foods, of which it is always a good idea to check the labels:

- olives

- crisps

- anchovies

- charcuterie

- saltine crackers

- snacks

Figure 11: How much sodium?

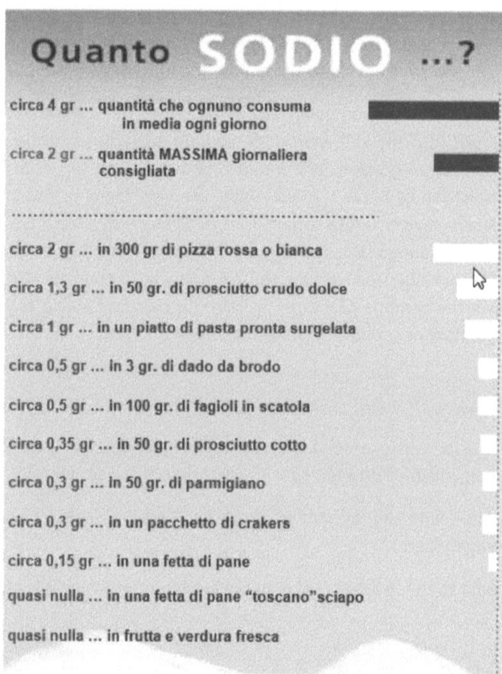

The figure above shows the amount of sodium that an Italian consumes on average each day (4 g) and the maximum recommended amount of sodium (2 g). The sodium content of some commonly consumed foods is also shown.

What happens if we decrease our daily sodium intake? The next figure is explanatory:

Figure 12: What Happens if We Decrease Daily Sodium Intake

Che cosa succede se ...	
Si riduce il sodio, cioè non si consuma più di 2 gr di sodio al giorno?	la pressione* cala di 6 -8 mm Hg
Si dimagrisce e si raggiunge il peso ideale?	la pressione* cala di 5-10 mm Hg ogni 10 Kg persi
Si segue una alimentazione ricca di frutta, verdura (riducendo grassi saturi e sodio)?	la pressione* cala di 8-14 mm Hg
Si svolge una attività fisica regolare (almeno 30 minuti al giorno di cammino a passo sostenuto) ?	la pressione* cala di 4-9 mm Hg

** I dati si riferiscono alla riduzione della pressione sistolica (massima). La diastolica (minima) cala di circa la metà.*

Sources: National Research Institute for Food and Nutrition

https://www.cuore.iss.it/prevenzione/pdf/sale_broch2pag.pdf

x. Food intolerances

Cellulite and water retention are sometimes favoured by foods that cause a negative response in our organism: for this reason, a food intolerance test might be a good idea, in particular the **cytotoxic test**, which is carried out with a blood test.

The cytotoxic test is based on the assessment of cellular damage, in particular of white blood cells, which occurs when a blood sample taken from the patient is placed in contact with the food to be tested (the list of foods tested is very long indeed).

xi. Anti-Cellulite Diet

The anti-cellulite diet should be very varied and complete, so as to ensure all the indispensable micronutrients, but also slightly low-calorie (especially if overweight), rich in fruit and vegetables, with a moderate amount of whole grains, low in fat and almost no added salt, as we have seen above.

In our daily diet, we should ban alcohol, limit coffee to a minimum, and avoid foods to which we are intolerant.

It may be useful to use *phlebotonic* supplements, i.e. supplements that protect the capillary walls:

- vitamin C
- bioflavonoids (contained in butcher's broom, Ginkgo Biloba, Centella asiatica)
- anticianosides (found mainly in bilberry)

Draining substances are certainly useful:

- artichoke
- sea oak (fucus vesiculosus)
- pilosella
- dandelion
- vitamin B6

Let's look at an example of a 1,500 Kcal/day anti-cellulite diet, with three main meals and a mid-morning snack.

EXAMPLE OF DIET	
BREAKFAST - 300 kcal • A cup of semi-skimmed milk • Barley coffee • Two rusks or three wholemeal biscuits • A citrus fruit juice	**AFTERNOON - 100 kcal** • An apple
MIDMORNING - 100 kcal • 2 kiwis or 3 California plums	**DINNER - 450 kcal** • 1 chicken breast or a slice of turkey • or 200 g lean fish (cod or sole) • A potato and a carrot • Lettuce salad: 100 g lettuce, 100 g tomatoes, 80 g radishes • One tablespoon of olive oil • 30 g wholemeal bread
LUNCH - 550 kcal • 80 g pasta or brown rice • One tablespoon of olive oil • 30 g pulses (chickpeas, peas, lentils ...) • 30 g wholemeal bread	**TOTAL kcal 1,500**

The above example of an 'anti-cellulite diet' is given for illustrative purposes only: the reader cannot and should not in any way understand it as a model diet to be applied and should consult qualified nutritionists. The reference source is in the public domain and can be found here:

https://massimospattini.com/la-cellulite/

Obviously, there is no such thing as a one-size-fits-all diet. Therefore, the previous example must be seen and interpreted as a starting point for understanding how one should structure one's diet to counter cellulite. There are so many specificities that it is impossible to generalise: just think of the variety of food intolerances, allergies, personal taste, one's morpho-biotype, the presence of any pathologies or inflammations, age, sex, the type of physical activity carried out during the day, the availability of food - which should be of high quality as far as possible, etc.

However, some general suggestions can be made.

It is important to include carbohydrates, proteins and fats whenever possible in meals (but not to overdo it with the anxiety and stress of having to introduce them at all costs in all meals of the day), as well as vegetables whenever meat, fish, rice and pasta are eaten.

It would be best to avoid eating a meat dish without vegetables, to avoid excess acidity in the body. Also, it is best to avoid eating different types of protein at the same meal, such as meat and cheese, eggs and meat, eggs and cheese, eggs and ham, etc., because they slow down digestion, as each type of protein needs particular enzymes that are activated under specific acidity conditions. In addition, milk casein tends to incorporate meat proteins, making them poorly digestible and resulting in putrefactive phenomena in the stomach.

Sources:

https://www.starbene.it/alimentazione/diete/cibi-acidi-alcalini-giusto-ph-dieta-antiacida/

https://www.metodo-ongaro.com/blog/nutrizione-combinazioni-alimentari-corrette

The main alkalising foods, rich in calcium, minerals and vitamins, are those that help remove the acidity introduced by foods such as industrial foods and meats.

Below is a non-exhaustive list of alkaline foods, easily found on the Internet:

Table 3: Alkalising Foods

ALKALISING FOODS	
Vegetables	* In particular, green leafy vegetables: spinach, chard, broccoli, cauliflower, celery * But also: cucumbers, onions, carrots, pumpkins, potatoes
Fresh Fruit	* In particular: apples, pears, bananas, grapes, pineapples, melons, mangoes, * But also: papaya, avocado, dates, strawberries, cherries, blueberries, plums, figs, dates and citrus fruits (especially lemon)
Dried Fruit	All, especially walnuts and almonds rich in omega 3
Cereals	Preferably whole grains, but not exclusively: millet, amaranth, brown rice, red rice, black rice, buckwheat and quinoa

It is well understood that, unless you have specific expertise in the field of nutrition, it is necessary to turn to qualified personnel: better to avoid DIY, or the advice of your friend, or your neighbour who found the magic diet in a fashion magazine....

By way of example only, below is a table with the most and least recommended foods to create a balanced diet to prevent, treat or manage cellulite (the source is the same as the one already mentioned in this section):

Table 4: Example of Recommended and Non-Recommended Foods

FOOD

RECOMMENDED	AVOID	STRONGLY DISCOURAGED
Fruit	Pastry shop	Sliced meats
Vegetables	Red meat	Canned foods
Olive oil	Dried fruit	Halls
Wholemeal bread	Coffee and tea	Dado
Pasta and brown rice	Butter	Salatini
Yoghurt	Margarine	French fries
Fresh cheeses	Whole milk	Fried
Skimmed milk	Ice cream	Hamburgers
Legumes	Eggs	Cream
Fish	Refined cereals	Besciamella
White meat	Matured cheeses	Mayonnaise
Organic fruit juices	Diet salt	Nutella
Organic vegetable	Wine	Chocolate
juices	Brown sugar	Fruit in syrup
Honey		Jams
		Refined sugar
		Snacks
		Fatty meat
		Spirits

IMPORTANT NOTE

Obviously, this list is entirely generic and must be adapted to the individual, depending on intolerances, the presence of any pathologies, physical activity, age, etc. What is said in this text about nutrition and supplementation is merely for illustrative purposes and must be read and evaluated with a critical eye: it cannot and will not in any way replace the skills of the professionals in charge of and qualified in nutrition, who are and remain the only reference figures in this field.

Finally, it is always good to remember that if a food is not recommended, it does not mean that it is banned from the table: a modest amount inserted in a correct dietary context can absolutely be consumed and give pleasure, without causing health problems.

xii. Acidifying and alkalinising foods

We have talked about acidifying and alkalinising foods, but we need to focus attention on a key concept: the pH of a food in itself does not determine its actual acidity within our body. The acidifying effect that foods can have in our bodies after being digested depends essentially on two factors:

1. The mineral **content:** minerals such as chlorine, iodine, bromine, fluorine, sulphur and phosphorous are negatively charged, resulting in an acidifying effect, while others, positively charged, such as calcium, magnesium and potassium, have an alkalinising effect.

2. **Protein content:** proteins, particularly if they contain sulphur amino acids, tend to form acids (organic acids formed when proteins are catabolised, i.e. broken down).

When food arrives in our stomach, it is 'welcomed' by the hydrochloric acid in it, which is even more acidic than the food itself, regardless of its starting pH. In fact, the hydrochloric acid brings everything to a pH close to 2: very acidic! After that, it all passes into the intestine, this time meeting the bicarbonate of the pancreatic juices, which buffers the acidity, making everything alkaline.

In conclusion: the acidity of a food has nothing to do with whether or not it is acidifying for the body.

Source: https://www.spaziosfera.com/blogdelnutrizionista/limoneacidificante.html

xiii.   The strange case of the lemon

The lemon is an extremely acidic fruit, with a pH close to 2, almost like that of the hydrochloric acid produced in our stomachs.

However, it is one of the most alkalinising foods in nature: in fact, it contains a lot of cations (positive ions), which neutralise the acids in our bodies. Thus, lemon is acidic, but it is not acidifying; in fact, it is even an excellent alkaliniser.

Sometimes we get the impression that lemonade burns or punctures the stomach: the stomach is more acidic than lemon juice, so it is just an impression, with no scientific basis.

A glass of cola drink, which contains orthophosphoric acid, is much more acidifying than a litre of lemonade...

Source: https://www.spaziosfera.com/blogdelnutrizionista/limoneacidificante.html

b.   Integration

Below, we will look at the main plant substances that provide valuable help in draining and eliminating excess fluid, decongesting the extracellular matrix and thus reducing the effects of cellulite. Many can be taken with a good diet, others can be supplemented appropriately. It is advisable to pay close attention to any allergies, intolerances, or pathological conditions, such as the use of medications, whose effect may be altered: always consult a doctor or nutritionist.

At the end of the section is a useful summary table, together with conclusions on 'anti-cellulite' food supplements. The above is essentially an excerpt from the following public page:

Main source:

https://massimospattini.com/drenanti-e-diuretici-naturali-per-contrastare-la-ritenzione-idrica/

i. Vitamin C

Vitamin C exerts antioxidant power, but also has a diuretic effect; it strengthens capillary walls and improves blood circulation.

The recommended dose is 1 g per day, which is easily achieved with a diet rich in plant-based foods. If supplements are needed to reach the indicated quota, it is preferable to take it sublingually: absorption through the oral mucous membranes is more efficient than with tablets.

ii. Escin

Escin is a plant compound obtained from the seeds, leaves and bark of the horse chestnut tree. It increases capillary resistance and venous tone. It decreases capillary permeability, improving oedema in the lower part of the body. Stimulates venous return: this is very useful in subjects suffering from heaviness and swelling of the legs, as well as cellulite. The recommended dosage is 100 mg per day.

iii. Diosmin

Diosmin is a bioflavonoid (an antioxidant substance found widely in nature) found in citrus fruits and birch leaves. It is mainly used for the treatment of haemorrhoids, due to its anti-inflammatory virtues, but is also used to promote the proper functioning of the veins (e.g. in cases of varicose veins, venous stasis in the lower limbs, gum or eye haemorrhages). In the treatment of venous stasis, it is effective in reducing oedema and draining excess extracellular fluid. Dosage can be as high as 300 mg / day, preferably divided into two separate intakes and away from meals.

iv. Centella asiatica

Centella asiatica is a herb used in traditional Chinese medicine. It favours the drainage of toxic substances in the body; it exerts an anti-inflammatory action in the tissues; it has a vascular-protective action; it improves the tone and elasticity of the walls of the arteries, veins and capillaries, thanks to the presence of proline and lysine, which stimulate the production of fibroblasts, the main constituents of the collagen of our blood and lymphatic vessels. Thanks to all these properties, it is particularly indicated in the treatment of venous insufficiency of the lower limbs, swelling, water retention and cellulite.

Centella asiatica supplements are available in the form of tablets or hydroalcoholic solutions, to be taken orally (holding them in the mouth for a few seconds to improve absorption). The recommended dose is 60 to 180 mg / day.

v. Melilot

Melilot is a plant that has been known since ancient Roman times, which increases venous tone and reduces capillary permeability; it has anti-inflammatory and diuretic properties; it reduces oedema; and it improves tissue oxygenation by promoting gas exchange in the capillaries. The recommended dosage ranges from 3 to 30 mg per day.

vi. Pilossella

Pilosella is an extremely popular plant with high diuretic and draining properties, very useful for treating cellulite, swollen ankles, oedemas and water retention; it promotes the excretion and outflow of bile, contributing to liver detoxification. Pilosella can be taken as capsules, at a dosage of 500 - 750 mg twice a day, away from meals, or as drops in mother tincture, at a dosage of 30 - 40 drops, twice a day, again away from meals.

vii. Dandelion

The root of the dandelion plant (also known as 'pisciacane' or 'dandelion', an extremely common plant in Italy), has a powerful draining action; it also has a depurative action, because it stimulates biliary, hepatic and renal function for the elimination of toxins and waste metabolites through faeces, urine and sweat. It stimulates the secretion of the glands of the digestive system (saliva, gastric and pancreatic juices, intestinal secretions), as well as the smooth muscles of the gastrointestinal tract, producing a mild laxative effect. It can be taken in tablets of 500 - 750 mg twice a day away from meals, or in drops of mother tincture diluted in a little water and sipped slowly, in quantities of 50 drops to be taken two to three times a day, again away from meals.

viii. Horsetail

Horsetail is the only fern plant belonging to the Equisetaceae family, also known as 'horsetails', which has survived from the Paleozoic era to the present day. It has capillary-protective properties; it is useful for the health and beauty of the skin; it has diuretic properties (useful for disposing of metabolites) due to its content of silica, calcium, magnesium, potassium, saponins and flavonic glycosides. It stimulates tissue repair, with a healing effect; it exerts a modest anti-cellulite effect, making the skin firmer and smoother to the touch and sight.

How to take it: as tablets in an amount of 190 mg / day, distributed several times during the day; or as a liquid extract in ethanol in an amount of 20 drops 3 times a day, between meals, sipping slowly.

ix. Natrum Sulphuricum and Thurya

Natrum Sulphuricum is very useful for reducing water retention. It is obtained from sodium sulphate, a derivative of salt and sulphuric acid, which takes the form of a white powder. It acts on the liver, kidneys, dysentery, joint rheumatism and periodic dermatological conditions.

Similar to Natrum sulfuricum we also find Thuja, of plant origin: they both belong to the homeopathic 'sycotic reactive' model (i.e. an imbalance of the immune system due to the action of several immunosuppressive factors) and provide homeopathic remedies against cellulite.

Method of intake: it is taken in granules. In homeopathy the taking of granules is different if they are used for chronic or acute problems:

- In the chronic phase it is usually recommended to take 5 granules at a time 3 times a day, away from meals;
- In the case of acute pathology, it is usually recommended to take the granules several times during the day at close intervals, up to 2 or 3 granules every one to two hours.

References for further reading:

https://www.cure-naturali.it/articoli/terapie-naturali/omeopatia/modelli-reattivi-omeopatia.html

https://www.reckewegcomics.com/omeopatia/rimedi-omeopatici/natrum-sulfuricum-omeopatia/

https://www.reckewegcomics.com/omeopatia/rimedi-omeopatici/thuja-occidentalis-rimedio-omeopatico/

https://www.tuttofarma.it/granuli-omeopatici/10312-boiron-natrum-sulfuricum-5ch-granuli-omeopatici-tubo-da-4gr.html

x. Collagen

Collagen is one of the most effective active ingredients for combating cellulite. It is a protein produced by our body and is found in the dermis, the thickest layer of our skin. However, the natural production of collagen starts to decline after the age of 22-23, so that the skin can lose its elasticity, tone and firmness. In addition, certain external causes can negatively affect its production, such as a diet with excess sugar. To effectively combat cellulite, and at the same time promote the skin's regeneration process, taking good amounts of collagen helps to restore elasticity, tone and firmness to the skin, reducing the orange-peel effect.

Collagen is found in quality meat and fish, but it is also necessary to minimise consumption of foods high in simple sugars, or processed meats (such as sausages).

Dietary supplements can help restore sufficient collagen levels to regenerate the skin: various types and concentrations are available on the market. It is considered a safe supplement as long as oral doses of no more than 2.5 mg per day are taken for up to 24 consecutive weeks. Allergic reactions are possible, particularly to collagen of bovine origin and in those allergic to eggs. In addition, the possible presence of other molecules (such as glucosamine) could trigger side effects such as nausea, heartburn, diarrhoea, constipation, drowsiness, headaches and skin reactions.

For more information:

https://www.humanitas.it/enciclopedia/integratori-alimentari/collageno-collagene-di-tipo-ii/

https://www.ncbi.nlm.nih.gov/pmc/articles/PMC4685482/

In the last reference above, an interesting 2015 research on the effects of collagen in the treatment of cellulite is reported. "The results obtained in this study showed that oral supplementation with specific BCP (bioactive collagen) over a period of 6 months resulted in a marked improvement in skin appearance in women suffering from moderate cellulite. Furthermore, the data showed the remarkable potential of BCP to improve the skin morphology of cellulite-affected areas, providing new evidence for the beneficial effects of BCP and postulating a new therapeutic strategy for the treatment of cellulite. "

xi. Hyaluronic acid

Hyaluronic acid is a molecule belonging to the group of glycosaminoglycans: these are substances produced by our body at the level of connective tissues (e.g. in joints and skin).

This molecule is able to bind numerous water molecules, giving turgidity and hydration to the tissues in which it is found. In fact, it keeps the skin moisturised and turgid, giving it a plumped and younger-looking appearance and removing wrinkles.

With advancing age, as early as our thirties, the body's production of hyaluronic acid gradually decreases and that which has already been formed tends to degrade, causing dehydration and loss of skin turgor, resulting in wrinkles.

In itself, therefore, hyaluronic acid is not strictly an anti-cellulite supplement; however, it can help restore tone and vigour to the skin, through a fuller, plumped-up appearance and the elimination of wrinkles.

Hyaluronic acid is often sold as a supplement together with collagen, in the form of capsules.

For more information:

https://www.humanitas.it/enciclopedia/integratori-alimentari/acido-ialuronico/

xii. Polyphenols (aronia juice)

This 2014 research

https://pubmed.ncbi.nlm.nih.gov/24433076/

showed that 100 ml per day of polyphenol-rich aronia juice for 90 days led 97 per cent of the subjects tested to a marked reduction in subcutaneous tissue thickness and oedema, with a clear beneficial effect on the condition of cellulite.

xiii. Other compounds

There are many other excellent supplements derived from plants, which are often part of extremely valuable compounds for their detoxifying and depurative properties, for example:

- bearberry

- milk thistle

- birch

- bromelain

- fennel

- aniseed

- melissa

For information purposes, the main supplements used to combat cellulite, swelling of the lower limbs, water retention and oedema are listed here.

These herbs and remedies are often available in the form of herbal teas, infusions and decoctions. However, the most effective absorption seems to be through drops or tablets, in which the active ingredients are more concentrated.

Some studies indicate that taking these compounds, through drops dissolved in a little water and sipped slowly, ensures better absorption through the mucous membranes.

Supplements formulated for drainage and diuresis usually have a mix of active ingredients, which results in a more powerful effect than using a single active ingredient.

It should also be borne in mind that some of these active ingredients can also have major side effects, so it is best to <u>AVOID DO-IT-YOURSELF, and to consult</u> specialised doctors and nutritionists.

<u>The indicated dosages are</u> also <u>for illustrative purposes only</u> and, of course, may vary depending on gender, age and pathology, as well as the type of mix of active ingredients. Let's take an example to clarify: the intake of milk thistle is absolutely not recommended in the presence of gallstones.

This section is also intended to provide information, so that we can understand for ourselves whether or not the supplement we are purchasing may have a positive effect on our body and on the management of cellulite, but under no circumstances can it replace the knowledge of the specialist treating a condition.

Using dietary supplements based on algae extracts to improve metabolism, pineapple and papaya to decongest and promote reabsorption, dandelion and birch to eliminate stagnant water from the tissues, gingko biloba and centella asiatica to tone the capillaries and improve circulation, as well as alpha-lipoic acid to improve metabolism (by decreasing fat, thus also fat in the buttocks), could be a valid strategy to follow, with the support of an expert in the field.

The following table provides a handy summary of the main active ingredients discussed in this section, with their dosage when used as the only active ingredient.

Ref: https://massimospattini.com/drenanti-e-diuretici-naturali-per-contrastare-la-ritenzione-idrica/

Table 5: Anti-cellulite supplements

ANTI-CELLULITE SUPPLEMENTS		
Vitamin C	Antioxidant; diuretic effect; strengthens capillaries; improves blood circulation	1 g/day (preferably sub-lingual and not tablets)
Escin	Increases capillary resistance and vein tone; improves oedema; stimulates venous return	100 mg /day

Diosmin	Anti-inflammatory; reduces oedema; helps drain excess fluid	300 mg / day, preferably divided into two separate intakes and away from meals
Centella Asiatica	Drains toxic substances; anti-inflammatory; vaso-protective; improves tone and elasticity of the walls of arteries, veins and capillaries	60 - 180 mg / die
Melilot	Increases venous tone and reduces capillary permeability; anti-inflammatory and diuretic; reduces oedema; improves tissue oxygenation	3 - 30 mg / die
Pilosella	High diuretic and draining properties; detoxifies the liver	* Capsules: 500 - 750 mg twice/day * Drops: 30 - 40 twice / die (!) Away from meals
Dandelion	Powerful draining; depurative; mild laxative	* Capsules: 500 - 750 mg twice/day * Drops: 50 two or three times / die (!) Away from meals
Horsetail	Protects capillaries; diuretic properties; healing; mild anti-cellulite (makes the skin smoother and firmer)	* Capsules: 190 mg / day (to be spread over several intakes) * Drops: 20 three times / die (sip slowly) (!) Away from meals
Natrum Sulphuricum and Thurya	Reduces water retention; acts on liver and kidneys	*Chronic phase: 5 granules at a time 3 times a day * Acute phase: up to 5 granules at a time every one to two hours a day (!) Away from meals
Collagen	Gives tone, elasticity and firmness to the skin	Capsules: 2.5 g per day x max. 24 weeks

c.   Exercise

Physical activity plays an essential preventive role with regard to cellulite, but it can also be effective in counteracting it, if not even in regressing it in the early stages of development, such as in the presence of oedema and slowed circulation; in the presence of fibrosis or sclerosis of the tissue, typical of the more advanced stages of the disease, training is not so effective, if used as the only weapon.

i. What are the most suitable workouts to combat cellulite?

Simplifying greatly, we could imagine muscles as being made up of two types of fibres: white or fast fibres, responsible for strength and instantaneous power, and red or slow fibres, intended for endurance (see figure below).

Figure 13: Muscle fibres

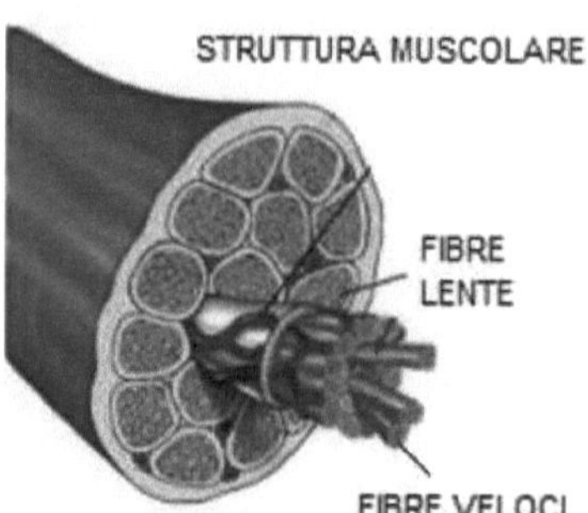

On average, women have more red fibres than men: these fibres mainly respond to aerobic metabolism, the metabolism that comes into play to burn fat using oxygen. Metabolism, in fact, is given by the composition of three energy systems:

- aerobic (with oxygen consumption)
- lactacid anaerobic (without oxygen consumption and with lactic acid production)
- alactacidic anaerobic (without oxygen consumption and without lactic acid production).

The effects of the three energy systems add up, depending on the intensity and duration of the effort. In the first seconds of exertion, the anaerobic alactacid metabolism comes into play, then the anaerobic lactacid metabolism, and finally only the aerobic metabolism remains active. It must be said, however, that the latter is always active and that is exactly what you are exploiting now, while reading this book.

An illustrative representation is shown in the diagram below:

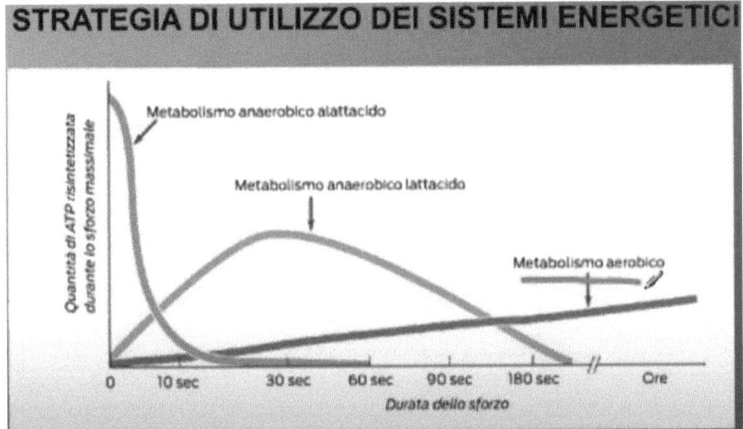

We will not go further into the technical explanation of these concepts, but will use them in this section.

As women have more red fibres (the slower, more endurance fibres) than men, they respond better to a higher volume (number of repetitions and sets) and load (number of exercises per weight used) of work. For the same reason, they respond better to continuous and regular work, and much less to HIIT (High Intensity Interval Training) type work. This training method is effective for reducing visceral fat (sub-abdominal fat, typical of men in the belly area) and much less so for subcutaneous fat (more prevalent in women). The latter, on the other hand, is consumed to a greater extent with slow and constant cross-country aerobic activity (e.g. cross-country walking, jogging, etc.).

The basic prerequisite of anti-cellulite training is the stimulation of circulation, both local and systemic (i.e. of the entire body), without producing too much lactic acid, which would contribute to increased local inflammation. However, a minimum production of lactic acid is to be sought, because the latter stimulates the production of GH, the so-called growth hormone, a protein that mobilises fat by stimulating lipolysis, i.e. allows fat to be used for energy purposes: this is exactly what we want to reduce cellulite.

Anti-gravity sports or physical activities are therefore recommended, such as swimming or water gymnastics, where in addition to the benefit of the physical activity itself, there is also the benefit of the massage provided by the water, which stimulates circulation.

Aerobic activity by means of a horizontal exercise bike is also recommended, which promotes circulatory return (the case with a traditional exercise bike is different, as illustrated in the next section).

Walking (or treadmill) at a brisk pace, or cross-country activities such as (slow) jogging, are highly recommended. In fact, the 'venous sponge' (see figure below) present in the sole of the foot is activated when walking, when the foot presses the sole to the ground: the capillary vessels in the sole of the foot are compressed and in this way push fluids upwards like a pump, giving rise to return circulation.

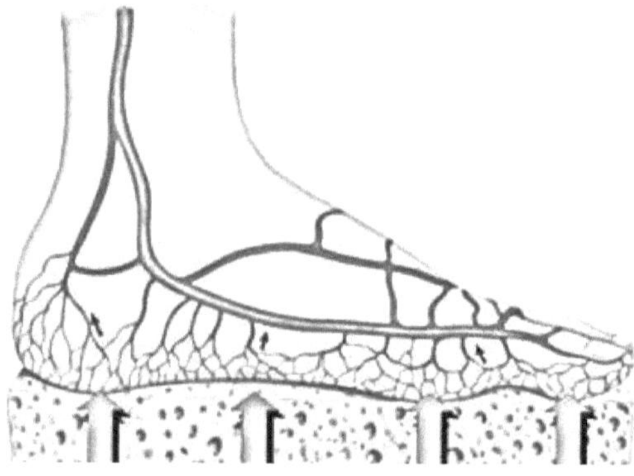

The case of running is different, in which the sponge is not activated in the same way, due to the mechanics of running itself. This is why running to combat cellulite is not recommended on various fitness websites: it is not particularly effective. However, it is not to be discouraged either, unless you have injuries, or particular health problems (herniated discs, heart problems, etc.), and/or joints. On the contrary: running can benefit the cardio-vascular system and help to 'take your mind off'.

For a walk to have a good effect in burning fat, it should last at least 40 - 50 consecutive minutes (preferably longer), with a heart rate that is between 65 - 75 % of the maximum heart rate (FCmax). There are a number of formulas for calculating FCmax: I suggest using an electronic device, such as a smartwatch, which can provide a reliable value from our biometric data.

Another extremely suitable workout is the so-called PHAT (Peripheral Heart Action Training), sometimes simply abbreviated to PHA. Hundreds of workouts of this type can be found on YouTube (just search for 'PHA training'), both for beginners and already trained individuals. It is a circuit training in which you alternate exercises for the upper body with others for the lower body. In this way, you work alternately on muscles that are far apart (upper and lower body), with cardio-type exercises (such as the horizontal exercise bike) in between: this promotes fluid circulation, preventing stagnation of liquids and metabolites (the products of metabolism), especially in the lower body. The lactic acid produced during the workout will also not stagnate in the areas affected by cellulite, avoiding an increase in acidity and therefore inflammation of the tissues: the well-being obtained will be considerable. In order to maximise the results, compatible with one's psycho-physical condition, it is suggested to set up a PHA type programme with a high number of repetitions and series using resistance (elastic bands or weights), lasting at least 30 minutes, but which can go up to 45 - 50 minutes. It is not advisable to exceed this threshold, to avoid accumulating too much lactic acid and impairing results. The only caution to be exercised is in choosing the type of PHA training according to the stage of cellulite: if we are in an advanced stage and heavily overweight, it may be preferable to train without too much jumping around. Here again, the assessment of an expert is crucial.

In general, it would be good to use a training method that evenly improves circulation in the areas most affected by cellulite.

Recently, a piece of equipment (hypoxi trainer) has been designed that can create localised depressurisation of the body to stimulate circulation mainly from the waist down. It consists of an exercise bike inserted inside a capsule that creates the depression. The user enters the capsule from the waist down, staying with the upper part of the body outside, as in the figure below:

Figure 16: Localised Depressurisation Training Equipment

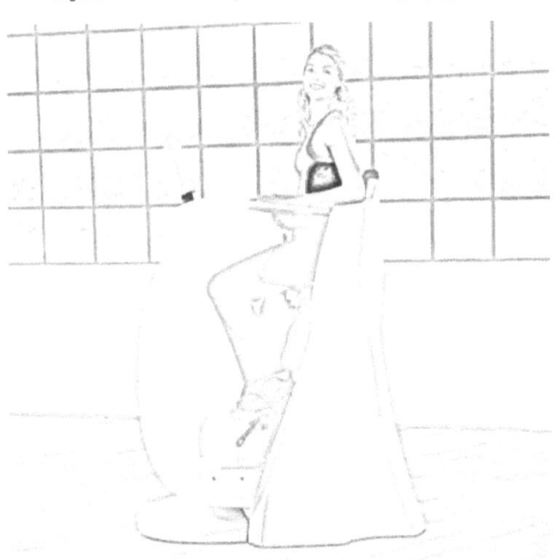

Source: https://www.euracom.it/it/corpo/20-hypoxi-trainer-s120.html

In this way, the body tries to counteract the lack of oxygen in the tissues affected by cellulite, thanks to the movement carried out in the presence of good oxygenation and circulation, and also mainly burns localised fat as an energy source.

An often debated topic is whether training with overloads (weights) improves or worsens cellulite. Training against resistance helps to build good muscle mass, at the expense of fat mass, and reduces water retention. From this point of view, therefore, it is good, but you have to know how to train, depending on your morpho-biotype and the conditions in which you find yourself. Multi-articular exercises with overloads (and not the 1 kg ankle supports...), which mainly stimulate the gluteal and femoral muscles, without forgetting the calves, which in turn act as a pump, both for the venous and lymphatic systems, should certainly be favoured. However, in the advanced stages of cellulite, some exercises may cause pain, due to poor local circulation: it is necessary to evaluate on a case-by-case basis, respecting the concept of progressiveness in training and, only as a last resort, excluding certain exercises, if one cannot do otherwise. Therefore, pay close attention to those who, without having even evaluated you, assert that exercises such as the squat are to be avoided, because they compress the veins and thus can create circulatory problems and worsen cellulite. Training, in fact, must be seen as a whole: by appropriately alternating the exercises as in the PHA method, the problem does not exist, not to mention that the seconds in which one is compressed during a squat session are not comparable to the minutes (hours...) of compression spent on a traditional exercise bike. The suggestion is to tackle the problem in its entirety, always relying on qualified and trained personnel. Only if you have the basics to understand these concepts, can you understand whether the person in front of you is a trained person or an improvised one...

ii. Some examples of PHA training with weights

Below are four examples of PHA weight training: two for beginners and two for intermediates (experts already know what to do...).

PHA 1 training - for beginners

Squat with Dumbbells: 10-12 repetitions

Lat Machine Pull Down: 10-15 repetitions

Push ups: 8-12 repetitions

Romanian Deadlifts: 8-12 repetitions

Reverse Crunch: 10-15 repetitions

PHA 2 training - for beginners

Overhead lifts with dumbbells: 10 repetitions

Sumo Squat with Kettlebell: 10-12 repetitions

Dumbbell rower: 8-12 repetitions per side

Crunches: 10-15 repetitions

Swing: 10-15 repetitions

Each of the two previous workouts consists of a circuit to be repeated 5 times, with an active rest (i.e. moving) of 2 minutes between circuits and 20 to 30 seconds between exercises, depending on your physical condition and the loads used.

PHA 3 training - intermediates

Sequence 1

Sumo squat with kettlebell: 10 repetitions

Overhead lifts with dumbbells: 8 repetitions

Standing Biceps Alternate Dumbbells: 8 reps per side

Sequence 2

Donkey Kick Machine (leg kicks backwards) or at the Cables: 15 repetitions per side

Dumbbell Lateral Raises: 8 repetitions

Standing Biceps Together Hammer Press: 8 repetitions

Sequence 3

Romanian Deadlifts with Barbell: 10 repetitions

Front lifts with dumbbells: 10 repetitions per side

Floor crunches: 15 repetitions

PHA Training 4 - intermediates

Sequence 1

Leg Curl: 10 repetitions

Lat Machine Pull Down Wide Grip: 10 repetitions

Triceps French Press Barbell on Flat Bench or with Rope Cables: 12-15 repetitions per side

Sequence 2

Forward Dumbbell Lunges: 10-12 repetitions per side

Low Pulley with Triangle: 12-15 repetitions

Triceps Push Down Rope to Cables: 12-15 repetitions

Sequence 3

Abductor Machine: 15-20 repetitions

Reverse Close Press Lat Machine: 8-10 repetitions

Reverse Crunch: 15-20 repetitions

Workouts 3 and 4 consist of 3 exercise sequences each. Each sequence must be repeated three times, resting actively for 1 - 2 minutes before repeating the sequence or moving on to the next one. There are no breaks between exercises in the sequence, other than the physiological ones to switch from one piece of equipment to another.

As a general rule, PHA training should be done three times a week for a beginner and four times a week for an intermediate, avoiding doing more than two consecutively, with no rest day in between.

A model training week for a beginner could be: Mon - Wed - Fri, or Mon - Thu - Sat.

A model training week for an intermediate could be: Mon - Tue - Thu - Fri, or Mon - Wed - Thu - Sat.

To a certain extent it is we who have to adapt to training, but to a large extent training has to adapt to our lifestyle and commitments, both work and personal, so that it becomes a good and pleasant habit and does not constitute an additional source of stress.

iii. What are the least suitable workouts to combat cellulite?

In addition to the HIIT workouts seen in the previous section, we can certainly count spinning or the traditional exercise bike as the least suitable for combating cellulite: in fact, the position assumed during the exercise creates an unfavourable angle between the torso and thighs and, as a result, compresses both the organs and the vessels inside the body, making circulatory return more difficult. It is better to use a horizontal exercise bike, where this angle is flattened and circulation is not hindered.

Running has no particularly positive effects on cellulite, because it does not significantly activate the 'venous sponge', as is the case with walking (see previous section).

As previously written, the fact that these workouts are less effective in combating cellulite does not mean that they should be banned.

iv. Let's recap: recommended and non-recommended workouts

We summarise in the following table the recommended workouts and those not recommended for preventing or regressing cellulite:

Recommended Workouts	Training Not Recommended
PHA	Running
Fast Walking	Traditional exercise bike
Jogging	Spinning
Swimming	HIIT
Physical Activity in Water	
Horizontal Exercise Bike	
Training with Overloads	
Hypoxi Trainer	

v. Exercises for swollen legs

In this section we illustrate two very simple and useful exercises to reduce swelling and pain in the legs and ankles by reducing fluid stagnation. This problem can occur for various reasons: with the summer heat, by wearing unsuitable footwear or clothing that is too tight, after a heavy workout, after too sedentary a job, or prolonged standing (hairdressers or shop assistants for example).

The first exercise is to lie on the floor or on the bed (as long as you are comfortable) and place a tennis ball under the sole of either foot. Then roll the ball under the bare foot, pressing it downwards: the important thing is that the supporting surface is rigid enough to provide a push upwards. This activates the venous sponge of the foot, reactivating circulation from the peripheral area (the foot) to the central area (the heart). One repeats the rotation of the foot for about a minute, then switches to the other foot. This exercise can be repeated 2 to 5 times per side, typically in the evening before going to bed, also daily, or whenever the need arises, such as after a leg workout:

Figure 17: Foot Rotation Over a Tennis Ball

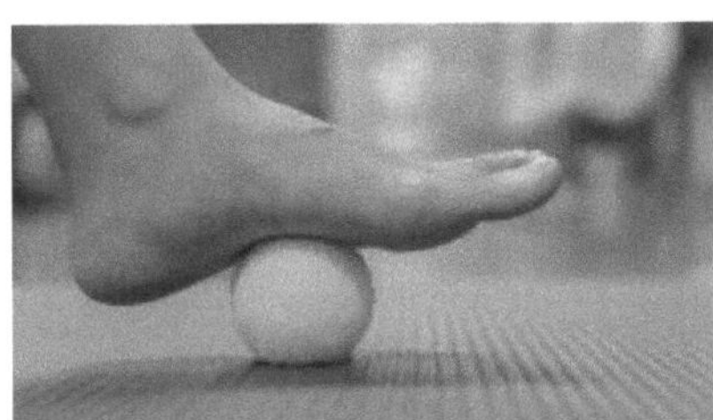

Another very effective exercise is to lie down on the floor and raise your legs in a square shape, leaning them against the wall, as in the figure below:

Figure 18: Squared Legs at the Wall

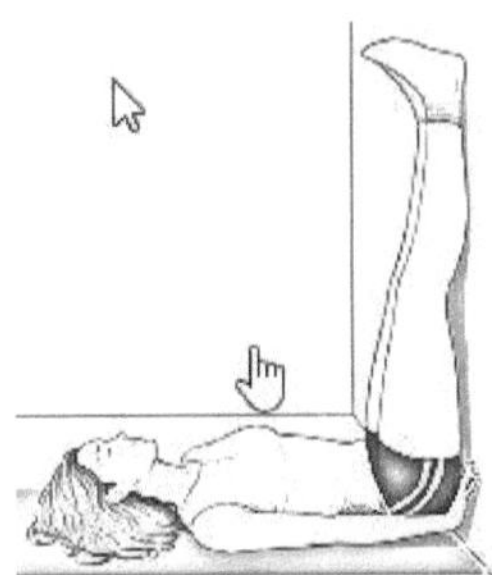

The simplest version of this exercise is to keep the legs elevated for a few minutes (e.g. 5 minutes), then lower them for a few seconds (e.g. 30 to 60 seconds) and repeat the exercise again. While lifting your lower limbs, you can try bending your ankles from top to bottom and vice versa, keeping your feet rigid: a bit like trying to accelerate and brake with the car pedals.

This will further stimulate venous return. You can also spread your legs apart and then return them to their original position, or bend them slightly to bring your knees towards your chest and then assume the squat position again.

A very interesting variation of the previous exercise consists of bending the knees slightly towards the chest and performing a walk on the wall, from bottom to top and vice versa. During the walk on the wall, the sole of the foot must be pushed well against the wall, activating the venous sponge.

Those who are better at coordinating movements can try this variation: lying with your back to the floor, legs raised and flexed at 90°, with the sole of the foot resting on the wall. In this position, perform thrusts towards the wall, contracting and decontracting, to stimulate the plantar venous sponge. The exercise can also be performed by placing a ball under the bare foot, compressing it to the wall.

Finally, I propose a simple routine to be performed when needed and if you have more time, followed by an explanatory image of the exercises to be performed:

Exercise (once per foot)	Duration
Foot rotation over a tennis ball (lying on the couch/bed es)	1 min

Circuit (repeat 3 to 5 times)	Duration
Overhead thrusts	40 sec
Butterfly Movement	40 sec
Alternating Forward Lunges	40 sec
Hammer toe leg crunches (move feet)	40 sec
ISO Squat	15 sec
Squat with Arm Push-Ups (burpees-like)	40 sec

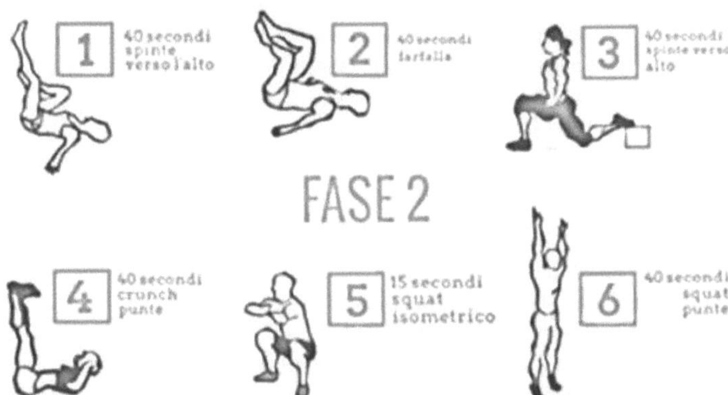

With the exception of the first exercise of rotating the foot over the tennis ball, the routine should be repeated three to five times for maximum benefit.

d.   Lifestyle

As we have seen in the previous sections, cellulite is a disease caused by several factors and therefore needs to be tackled across the board. Lifestyle, understood in the broadest possible sense, is one of the main causes of this disease.

i. Stress even at the table

Stress in excess leads to alterations of various kinds: irritability, loss of sleep or its quality, digestive problems and possible gastro-intestinal inflammation. All of this alters our homeostasis, i.e. our psychic and hormonal balance, resulting in a continuous rise in the stress hormone, cortisol, which in turn lowers our immune defences, with a further increase in inflammatory states. By not resting well, our body cannot recover and the production of hormones is completely out of sync. So if we already have a situation of localised inflammation due to the presence of cellulite, excessive stress will only make it worse. Obviously we are not talking about an acute stress phase, but a chronic stress phase, which lasts for a long time.

We also avoid stress when we eat. In fact, food, once ingested, is also conditioned by external factors. Let us therefore avoid distractions at the table: getting up often to check the pots and pans on the cooker that are on, answering our smartphones or phones, reading or watching TV, etc. If we are in company, we avoid topics that can cause tension...

Let us remember to chew well, especially when we eat carbohydrates, especially complex ones, such as pasta, bread, pizza, potatoes, etc. In fact, the first digestion of these foods takes place in the mouth, thanks to enzymes present in our saliva (such as amylase). We take the time to eat well: the sight, smell, sound of food and even the thought of food produce a series of stimulatory signals directed to the central nervous system. From there, other stimuli reach the stomach, increasing the secretion of gastric juice, preparing us for digestion. Mealtime is a time of joy and satisfaction for ourselves: let us enjoy it, take the time and care necessary to benefit from it.

ii. How to limit stress?

First of all, we need to identify the main sources of stress: work, family, friends, illness, negative thoughts, everything can contribute to us losing balance. The first step is to understand what is creating our anxiety, stress and/or nervousness and what are its causes.

The second, is to understand what we can do to eliminate the source of stress that is gripping us. If, for example, we are hanging out with friends who cause us discomfort, or who influence our lives in a negative way, we must take note of this and change our attitude towards them. We can try dialogue in the first instance, trying to address the problem in a direct but polite manner. If that is not enough, we have to take much stronger measures, such as limiting the presence of these people in our existence, or even closing our relations with them for good. This is an extreme solution, but sometimes it is the only one possible, so that we do not pollute and deteriorate our lives. These people who are 'toxic' to our existence can be friends, lovers, family members, acquaintances... The closer the relationship, the more difficult it will be for us to face the situation and accept it for what it really is. However, the first person to love is ourselves: this is not an act of selfishness, but a firm and decisive stance, not cancelling ourselves out to please others, in favour of respect and love for ourselves, which we deserve just as much as those around us. We must not let ourselves be trampled on in our feelings, emotions, ideas, or even physically by anyone: of course, neither must we do this to others. These considerations may seem trivial, but how many of us really have the courage to take care of ourselves, at the cost of being alone, at least initially, without being trapped in ties and constraints dictated by our culture, the teaching we have had from our families and the society in which we live? How many of us are really so strong as to be able to free ourselves from the superfluous that creates slavery, such as the lust for possessing objects, which in turn make us slaves to their custody and maintenance, sometimes even making us invisible to others?

If a source of stress cannot be eliminated, then we must manage it, limit it. For example, our wonderful mind often asks us recurring questions that are impossible to answer, creating anxiety: what will happen in the next few years? Will I manage to find the love of my life, a job and start a family? What would have happened if I had made a different decision that day? And if I became ill, what would happen to my children? It really bothered me the way my husband looked at his colleague yesterday: is he cheating on me with her? When these thoughts pop into our heads, returning in waves, nagging and hammering, digging, like woodworms, imaginary furrows in our minds, we are shaken, restless: soon anxiety assails us and we begin to live badly, losing our tranquillity. Again, the first step is to be able to recognise them; then learn to let them flow freely, not being afraid of them, but not giving them importance either. We should behave as outside observers: the thought presents itself, I take note of it, without expressing any opinion about it, I let it move away from me, a bit like observing, from the bank of a river, the trunk of a tree floating, carried away by the current. As we give importance to these thoughts, they take on greater relevance and, not having concrete answers to provide, our brain continues to propose them to us in an insistent and nagging manner: that is why we must recognise them and let them flow without passing judgement on them, whatever they may be. If I do not dwell on them, they cannot materialise and therefore cannot harm me. It sounds easy, but it takes a lot of practice to become aware.

iii. Breathing and meditation

For millennia, man has developed techniques to manage stress: there are various forms of meditation, as we have often seen on TV, or in training courses. They are all based on posture and breathing: respecting our body, giving it the dignity it deserves, is an essential point. Even the rosary practised by Catholic Christians can be seen as a form of meditation, beyond the religious component.

Meditation uses a certain form of breathing, which gives rhythm and concentration. The mind tends to wander, behaving like a monkey jumping from one branch to another in the jungle: it is its way of doing, acting, manifesting. We take note of this and, during meditation, thanks to a guiding voice, we bring our attention back to the object of meditation itself.

What are the objects of meditation? Firstly, the breath, which is life. Then a part of our body, such as a foot or a leg: we should not be surprised, rediscovering ourselves is fundamental; what will surprise us is learning how little we know about ourselves. In a second step, we will turn our attention to our being within nature, to understand its harmony and how we are part of it, having rediscovered it. Finally, we will learn how to meditate in any circumstance, such as during a walk or a bike ride, rediscovering the art of wonder.

I always recommend starting to learn some basic breathing techniques that help you relax and manage stress: they are simple forms of self-knowledge and meditation. Breathing is meditating... Some of the easiest breathing techniques to use are: square breathing, Dr Andrew Weil's 4-7-8 breathing, all the way to Wim Hoff's guided breathing. Some of these techniques can also be easily used throughout the day, such as at work, at home, or in the park. All the techniques mentioned can be easily found on the Internet, especially on Youtube.

References:

https://www.youtube.com/watch?v=4-YaTaIEqWI

https://www.youtube.com/watch?v=EUpKfdIMPNU

https://www.efficacemente.com/sonno/metodo-4-7-8/

iv. No smoking, no alcohol

Smoking does not cause cellulite, but it can make it worse, making it more visible. In fact, it causes premature ageing of the skin by reducing the ability of skin cells to retain moisture. Moisturised skin tissue results in more relaxed and toned skin, with fewer wrinkles. As the venous circulation is more fatigued and slowed down due to smoking, there is less oxygenation in the blood, as a result the cells will struggle to expel excess fluid, causing water retention.

Alcohol strains the microcirculation, promotes cellular ageing and broken capillaries.

Spirits, particularly cocktails, are the most harmful, both because of the percentage of alcohol they contain and the amount of sugar. Excess sugar turns into excess calories, which then become fat accumulation. Beer and wine have less damaging effects on water retention, as they have a lower percentage of alcohol than spirits. Therefore, during a dinner with friends, if you just can't help drinking, prefer a glass of red wine or a glass of beer, which not only contain less alcohol, but also less sugar.

v. Physical activity in the open air

The benefits of the sun on our bodies are many and well known. We summarise below those that have the greatest impact in combating cellulite.

Exposure to the sun encourages the production of:

-   Serotonin during the day, the so-called 'feel-good hormone

-   Melatonin in the evening, a hormone that 'decreases stress' and facilitates sleep

-   Vitamin D

Ultraviolet rays (in particular the UV-B frequency band) have the energy to transform part of the cholesterol, present between the lipid layers of our skin, into vitamin D precursors, which the liver and kidneys then transform into the hormone vitamin D. It is difficult to obtain vitamin D outside the summer season in our latitudes, which is why supplementation, preferably daily, is often required.

Sunlight regulates the sleep-wake cycle, thanks to the alternation of night and day: this is true if we do not wear sunglasses all the time, otherwise this effect is cancelled out. It also promotes muscle relaxation and joint mobility, thanks to the heat it emits through infrared rays. Finally, it improves acne, psoriasis, certain forms of dermatitis and eczema, as well as tanning the skin (by increasing melanin production).

In summer, in our latitudes, one must expose oneself to sunlight sensibly to avoid damage to collagen and skin tissue, leading to sunburn, premature skin ageing and wrinkles. UV rays can damage the skin's DNA and promote the formation of moles and even tumours, such as melanoma.

The benefits provided by exposure to the sun cannot be obtained with artificial light, except to a small extent with suitably calibrated UV lamps. The sun provides a good mood, supplies us with vitamin D, which is very useful for a myriad of processes, including anti-inflammatory ones, regulates the sleep cycle: just 20 to 30 minutes of exposure to sunlight is enough to produce melatonin and lower stress.

That is why it is so important to be outdoors whenever we can. If, in addition, we are also able to do adequate physical activity outdoors, we will gain a double benefit for the whole body and, ultimately, also for cellulite.

Healthy skin and a body in good general condition also help to improve, if not eliminate, the cellulite problem.

vi. Sedentary lifestyle

We have seen in previous sections how important it is to be outdoors whenever we can, as well as how important it is to move around, walking to activate the venous pump in the soles of our feet.

However, the lives of many of us are mostly sedentary and indoors: office work, long journeys while sitting in cars or on means of transport for commuting, etc. The end result is to find ourselves exhausted in the evening, lounging on the sofa watching TV.

Our social evolution has been at the expense of our psycho-physical health: we must take note of this. Since we are unlikely to revolutionise our society in a time compatible with our earthly existence, what we can concretely achieve is the introduction of a series of small changes in our lives, aimed at limiting sedentariness as much as possible. Let us remember, in fact, that sitting for a long time causes compression of the veins and capillaries, worsening the microcirculation in the areas affected by cellulite; likewise, clothing and posture can have negative effects, compressing our sub-abdominal organs, in turn worsening local circulation. Our footwear may not be suitable for activating the venous pump in our feet. We may also not be drinking or eating properly, as well as smoking or exaggerating with alcohol.

How can we change our habits?

Let's start with making small and simple daily improvements. If I have a water dispenser at work to quench my thirst, I can get a glass or metal bottle and fill it up to half. When the water is finished, I will have to get up to go and refill it. If I do not remember to drink, because I am too busy with my work worries, I can set a reminder to drink at least one glass of water every two hours. I could adopt a similar strategy to get up from my chair at least once every hour, for a few minutes: in this little break, I could take advantage of it to take a little walk through the office corridors (if I can't go outside) and do some stretching, at least in my wrists, ankles and neck. When sitting, I might remember not to cross my legs and to rotate my ankles often, as well as my wrists.

These are small tricks to be repeated daily, but they bring immediate benefits, also to our level of mental concentration.

Surely the most valid suggestion is to include walking whenever possible: to make the journey to work, or at least part of it, or on weekends in the open air, such as in parks, at the seaside, at the lake, in the woods, in the hills or in the mountains, as long as it is in nature, away from polluting and stressful sources.

Move, move and more move!

Let us rediscover the pleasure of being in the midst of nature: we will be amazed at how pleasant it is to breathe, feeling the air pass through our nose, our mouth, our oesophagus to reach our lungs and fill them with oxygen. We will be pleasantly and naturally amazed by the sensations we will receive and our body will awaken from its torpor, rejuvenating, like spring.

e.   Aesthetic and Therapeutic Treatments

Cellulite must be attacked with all the tools at our disposal. A number of aesthetic and therapeutic treatments, provided by specialised centres and personnel, come to our aid: we will look at the main ones below. The following sections on aesthetic treatments have been written with the valuable support of Simone Serafini, of the Serafini Medical Centre in Follonica (GR):

https://www.fisioterapiaserafini.it/

i. Pressotherapy

Pressotherapy consists of exerting a certain amount of mechanical pressure on the areas affected by cellulite, using a special device, which allows the drainage of liquids. One is wrapped in a kind of inflatable blanket, which rhythmically compresses and decompresses the covered areas. The following image is explanatory:

Figure 20: Pressotherapy

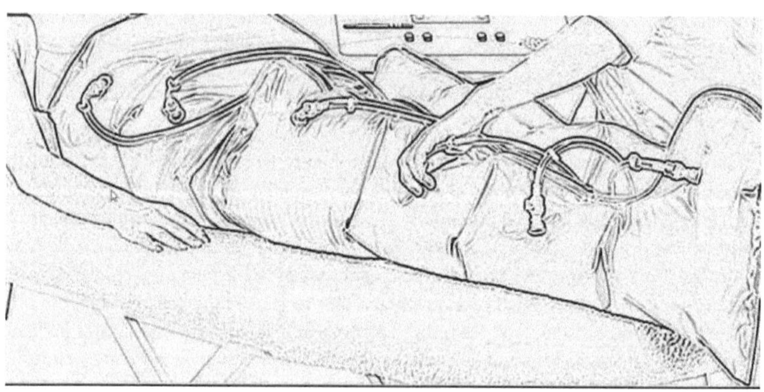

Pressotherapy sessions typically last between 15 and 50 minutes and the sequence of massage, compression and decompression (by 'inflating and deflating' the suit in which you are wrapped), varies between 10 and 20 cycles. One must be fasting to undergo the therapy.

Usually, 2 or 3 sessions per week are carried out, for a cycle of 8 to 12 sessions, to be repeated over the year as required. On average, appreciable results start to be seen as early as the fourth/fifth session.

It should be specified that mesotherapy does not solve cellulite, but the skin imperfections associated with it.

For further information:

https://www.formapro.it/pressoterapia-funziona-pro-contro-trattamento/

https://www.melarossa.it/bellezza/pressoterapia/

ii. Mesotherapy

Mesotherapy consists of injecting medication under the skin through tiny needles to help the process of eliminating excess fluid while toning the skin.

The drug solution usually contains amino acids, minerals, enzymes, hormones and vitamins, which are injected into the middle layer of the skin: the dermis (see figure below). The injected solution is specially prepared for the person receiving it; therefore, it is essential to contact qualified personnel to avoid even serious problems in the event of an allergy to certain components of the drug.

At least 30 minutes before inserting the needles, an anaesthetic cream is applied to the area of interest: the patient will not feel any discomfort.

Figure 21: Skin layers

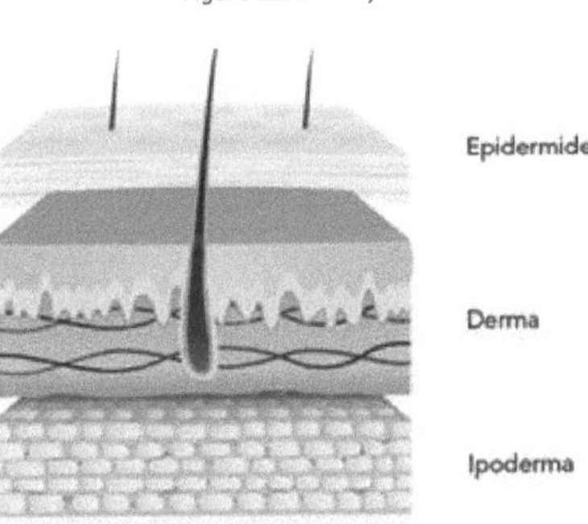

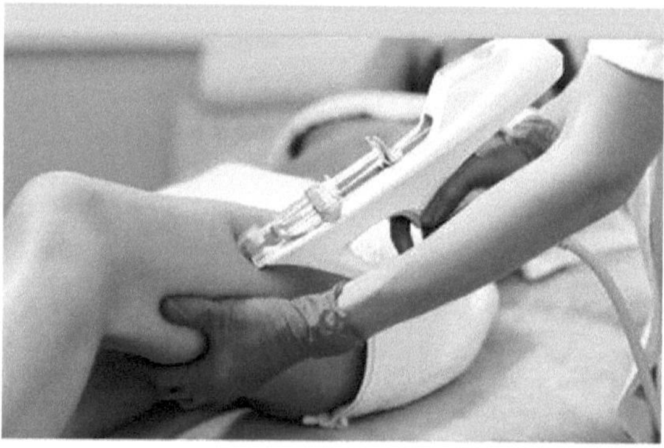

The number of mesotherapy sessions depends on the extent of the problem to be solved. For the treatment of cellulite associated with mild venous insufficiency of the lower limbs, one session per week for 8-10 weeks is usually sufficient, followed by a maintenance of one session every 15 days. After a mesotherapy session, it is a good idea not to do any massage or lymphatic drainage sessions or sports activities for at least one day: the injected product should remain in the thickness of the skin for as long as possible, thus allowing a better therapeutic effect.

It should be specified that mesotherapy does not solve cellulite, but the skin imperfections associated with it.

For more information:

https://www.humanitas.it/news/mesoterapia-cose-e-come-si-svolge/

https://www.vanityfair.it/gallery/mesoterapia-toglie-la-cellulite-dai-glutei-la-nostra-indagine-massaggi

iii. Ultrasound cavitation

Ultrasound cavitation is a process in which ultrasound waves are transferred to areas of the body affected by cellulite. Ultrasound leads to the rupture of the membrane of fat cells, exploiting the physical principle of cavitation. As they pass through a liquid, the waves create pressure changes, forming microbubbles in the fat cells, which implode after a short time, damaging the cell membrane. The fat contained in the cell escapes, entering the bloodstream and reaching the liver and kidneys, where it is finally disposed of. The treatment also has beneficial effects on the drainage of body fluids, alleviating cellulite and reactivating the peripheral circulation.

In technical terms, cavitation stimulates lipolysis, i.e. the decrease in the volume of fat cells, and lipoclase, i.e. the destruction of the fat cells themselves.

Ultrasound cavitation is suitable for reducing fat pads located in areas of the body that are not too large, while it is not recommended for severely overweight people, as it only acts on localised fat deposits. For this reason, it is often used to eliminate localised excess fat after liposuction or abdominoplasty operations.

To optimise fat dissolution, a physiological solution could be injected before ultrasound application.

A gel is applied to the treated area to help the ultrasound penetrate the adipose tissue.

A session usually lasts 20 to 30 minutes. The number of sessions varies depending on the extent and area to be treated, as well as on the state of hydration of the body, and other parameters assessed during the aesthetic doctor's examination. Sessions are generally performed at intervals of about 10 days.

Once the desired results have been achieved, maintenance sessions a few months apart may be recommended.

References: https://www.gloriamisasimedicinaestetica.it/tecniche-di-cavitazione-ultrasonica/

Figure 23: Ultrasound cavitation

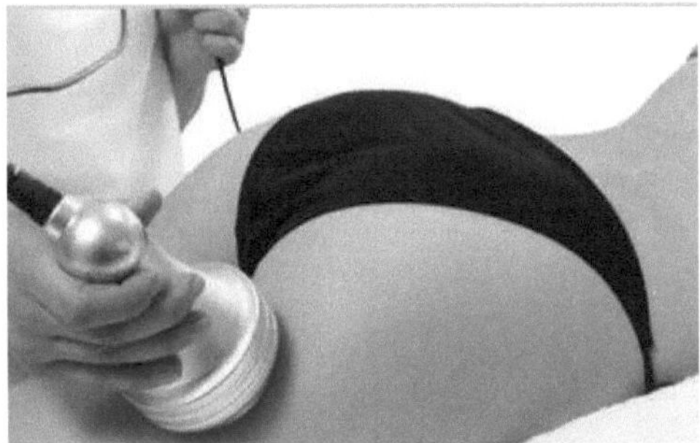

iv. Tecar therapy

Tecar therapy is a technique that stimulates energy within biological tissues, activating natural reparative and anti-inflammatory processes. It increases metabolic activity, boosting ATP production and thus speeding up cellular repair. It also improves blood circulation and lymphatic drainage, thanks to the vasodilation induced by the heat produced: this allows better oxygenation of tissues and reabsorption of oedemas. The advantage of tecar therapy, compared to other energy therapies, is that the energy is produced inside the cells (under stimulation of the equipment from outside), so it is also possible to affect deep layers.

It is a safe technique and is not at all invasive, let alone painful.

Tecar therapy stimulates the microcirculation, draining excess fluid and acting on inflammation; it increases the deep vascularisation, increasing the internal temperature, thus stimulating the natural enzymatic processes, which help dissolve fat nodules, the cause of the so-called 'orange peel effect'.

Usually, the minimum time for an anti-cellulite treatment is about 30 minutes, with a frequency of 2 sessions per week for the first 2 weeks, and one session per week for the next 4 weeks. However, the frequency of sessions can vary, even a lot, depending on the medical assessment of the individual patient who decides to undergo this treatment.

For those curious about technology: from a physical point of view, Tecar (Capacitive and Resistive Energy Transfer) is an acronym for both capacitive and resistive energy transfer.

Energy transfer in capacitive mode is carried out through an electrode, which is placed in contact with the patient's skin and covered with an insulating material (Teflon, ceramic or similar). The higher frequency current flows mainly through the muscles and soft tissues in general, which are rich in fluid, i.e. the most capacitive parts of the human body.

The resistive system, on the other hand, uses an electrode without any coating: it is easily recognisable because only the metal (steel) is visible on the surface without any kind of covering, as is the case with the capacitive electrode. The lower frequency current flows mainly through bones, joints, ligaments, tendons, i.e. the most resistive parts of the human body.

The following image is explanatory:

Figure 24: Tecar therapy

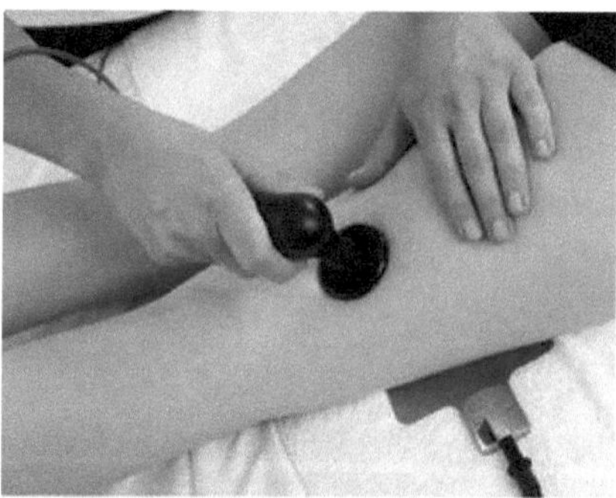

For more information:

https://fisioterapiadonna.it/tecar-per-cellulite/

v. Laser therapy

Laser therapy (also called laser lipolysis) is a painless and minimally invasive technique to heal cellulite and localised fat deposits. A thin optical fibre - about 1 mm in diameter - connected to a laser is inserted into the fatty area to be treated through a very small incision under local anaesthesia.

Figure 25: Laser therapy (laser lipolysis)

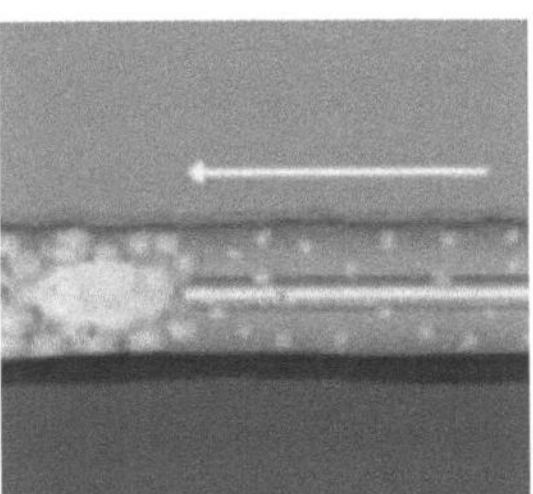

The thermal effect of the laser causes the fat to liquefy, turning into an oily substance, which is sucked out. The heat generated by the laser stimulates the fibroblasts (connective tissue cells) to produce more collagen and elastin (proteins that give the skin its elasticity and firmness) for up to a month after the procedure. Consequently, in the days following the treatment there is a progressive improvement and remodelling of the treated area, which becomes firmer and more toned in a short time.

The duration of a session depends on the stage and type of cellulite to be treated: typically 30 to 60 minutes. One treatment may be sufficient.

After the treatment, the patient must wear a restraining sheath, invisible and easily washable, for a month. The incisions do not require stitches and heal in a few days: small plasters are applied. However, this is a real operation, so absolute rest is recommended for the next 48 hours, but by the third day it is possible to return to work and walk without any problems.

The results obtained with this technique are definitive. Any weight gain will not be a problem because the fat will be distributed evenly.

It is essential to seek the services of experienced medical specialists, who operate in a sterile medical-surgical environment.

For more information:

https://www.medicitalia.it/blog/medicina-estetica/564-laser-lipolisi-l-ultima-frontiera-contro-la-cellulite.html

vi. Liposuction, Ultrasonic Liposuction, Liposculpture and
Microliposculpture

Liposuction, Ultrasonic Liposuction, Liposculpture and Microliposculpture are technically very similar procedures, because they are types of liposuction: however, they differ, depending on the area to be treated and the purpose they serve.

Liposuction is indicated for treating medium to large accumulations of cellulite. Cannulas of 5-6 mm in diameter, i.e. of large calibre, are used to remove excess fat accumulations. However, it is not an aesthetic procedure, i.e. it is not intended to eliminate cellulite, but to remove disabling excess fat accumulations.

Ultrasonic liposuction is indicated for treating medium to large fat deposits. Cannulae with a diameter of 4-5 mm are used. There is a certain risk from the ultrasound (see ultrasound cavitation), and it usually has limited effectiveness against cellulite blemishes.

Liposculpture is a genuine **cosmetic surgery** procedure suitable for removing medium to small cellulite accumulations. Cannulas with a diameter of 3-4 mm, i.e. medium to small, are used. Unlike liposuction, it restores aesthetic harmony to the shape of the treated area and allows cellulite to be eliminated.

Microliposculpture is a **cellulite-resolving** procedure, which is indicated for treating small fat accumulations. Cannulas with a diameter of 1-2 mm are used, i.e. very small.

All operations are performed under anaesthesia (local or general), so post-operative recovery needs to be assessed on a case-by-case basis. In addition, the cosmetic surgeon will have to correctly calculate the volume to be suctioned, avoiding problems of emptying the area, which could even lead to an adhesion effect between the surfaces, by carefully choosing the fat to be removed.

For more information:

https://www.dottordileo.com/liposuzione-liposcultura-microliposcultura-eliminare-la-cellulite/

vii. Lymphatic Drainage Massage

Lymphatic drainage massage has the task of draining liquids from areas of the body where they are stagnant, to promote their expulsion and induce deflation. In fact, the treatment acts directly on the lymphatic system, contributing to the disposal of **excess toxins that are** harmful to the body.

The lymphatic system is a collection of thin vessels (called lymphatics) that connect different organs, such as the bone marrow, tonsils, thymus, spleen and lymph nodes. In fact, it constitutes our body's defence system, as it drains excess fluid and toxins. In a way, it is like a parallel system to the cardiovascular system.

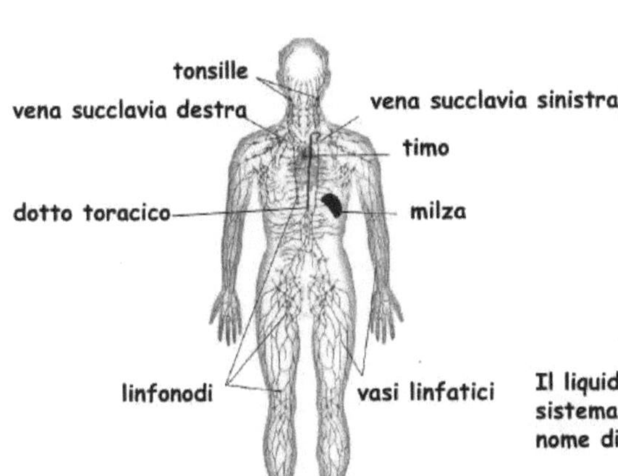

Figure 26: Lymphatic system

Along the lymphatic pathways we find the lymph nodes, peripheral organs responsible for the creation of lymphocytes, i.e. white blood cells that are responsible for the elimination of hostile microorganisms. The lymph, unlike the blood, is not propelled by cardiac activity, but by the action of the muscles which, by contracting, act as a pump.

The lymphatic drainage massage stimulates the lymphatic system, promotes the circulation of liquids to the lymph nodes and the toxin disposal process.

Water retention is an accumulation of fluid that causes unpleasant swelling, especially on the thighs, stomach and buttocks. There are various causes, as we have already seen: overweight, too little or too much physical activity, excessive stress, bad eating habits and/or lifestyle. To ascertain the presence of water retention, it is a good idea to consult a doctor, who will prescribe a urine test. However, you can also proceed with a small manual test, pressing your thumb on the affected area for about two seconds: if, after removing your finger, the imprint still remains clearly visible for a few seconds, you most likely have water retention.

viii. Mud Massage

The treatment based on warm mud, which envelops the body like a blanket, has a direct action on localised imperfections in the most critical areas, such as the thighs, hips and buttocks. The thermal mud exerts a draining and slimming action, activating the metabolism and eliminating toxins and impurities, thus improving the possible presence of cellulite.

Mud is often mixed with essential oils to promote deep tissue purification; Fucus and Laminaria algae, on the other hand, promote a lipolytic action.

The thermal mud treatment is ideal for all types of cellulite, stimulating lipolysis and tissue drainage. It is mainly practised in winter, as it is applied warm to the areas of interest.

The operator's subsequent massage stimulates the circulation, acting on the stagnation of liquids, as well as instilling a feeling of well-being and general relaxation, smoothing the skin and reducing orange peel skin.

The treatment lasts between 50 and 60 minutes and can be repeated several times a week, depending on the advice of the experienced practitioner. It is contraindicated in the presence of thyroid disorders.

References: https://amedeolucente.it/news-medicina-oftalmologia.asp?codice=10250

ix. Anti-cellulite creams

We have already extensively analysed the main supplements useful for combating cellulite: in this section, we will easily understand their working principles.

The following is a non-exhaustive list of the most common plant extracts contained in an anti-cellulite cream:

- **Algae**: draining, energising and lipolytic.

- Caffeine: caffeine stimulates circulation and promotes lipolysis, i.e. the melting of fat cells. However, this only occurs with topical use (i.e. on the skin): drinking coffee does not promote circulation, nor does it improve cellulite.

- **Carnitine**: is an amino acid useful for burning fat for energy and strengthening skin cells.

- **Centella asiatica**: is a plant capable of stimulating fibronectin, a protein that helps to strengthen blood vessel walls and prevent swelling and heaviness in the legs and ankles.

- **Escin**: is an extract that increases capillary resistance and reduces capillary permeability, reducing water retention and swelling, promoting capillary circulation and reducing heaviness in the legs.

- **Flavonoids:** natural compounds with protective action on capillaries and microcirculation, used in treatments to stimulate subcutaneous circulation.

- **Ginkgo biloba**: a complex of active ingredients, very rich in bioflavonoids, with beneficial properties on the circulatory system.

- **Retinol:** a derivative of vitamin A, it brings many benefits to the skin from an aesthetic point of view, as it smoothes it and improves its appearance.

- **Saponins:** increase the resistance of capillaries, decreasing their permeability and promoting fluid reabsorption.

- **Vitamin C:** essential for collagen synthesis, has anti-inflammatory and antioxidant properties

Anti-cellulite creams are very effective in improving the appearance of the skin by smoothing and toning the affected area. They do not combat cellulite directly, but they are certainly very helpful in reducing the orange-peel appearance of the dermis.

The cream should be applied over long periods by massaging the skin with circular movements to reactivate the circulation under the skin. The application must be constant and long-lasting: it can take up to several months to see an appreciable result.

After reading this section, when you buy an anti-cellulite cream, simply by reading its active ingredients you will be able to understand whether or not it will help you.

References: https://www.tuttogreen.it/guida-alla-crema-anticellulite/

8. Let us dispel some false myths

In this section we will dispel some false myths that have been circulating for years.

i. Cellulite is not fat

How many times have we heard that cellulite is merely an accumulation of fat? By now, it should be clear that this statement is an oversimplification.

In the same way, it could be argued that the brain is just fat, given its chemical composition.

Adiposity is an increase in the volume of fat cells (adipocytes). If it affects the whole body, it is general adiposity, resulting in overweight; if it only affects certain areas, it is localised adiposity. In both cases, it is an enlargement of fat cells.

Cellulite is an alteration of the skin tissue, which starts from the adipose layer (the deepest one) and reaches the upper layers: dermis and epidermis. Thus, it is primarily a localised inflammatory state, due to the causes already analysed in this text, which, as it worsens, can become real cellulite, with local fat accumulation, often due to poor microcirculation and excess calories in the diet.

This explains, moreover, why some very skinny girls on a strict low-calorie diet have cellulite. In fact, it all often stems from poor microcirculation: the causes are essentially genetic, but can be emphasised by wearing clothes that are too tight, as well as by too tight and high heels, a sedentary lifestyle or too many hours spent standing in the same position, incorrect posture, inadequate nutrition and hydration, smoking, etc. In the early stages there is a stagnation of liquids between the cells, due precisely to the poor local circulation, which does not allow a correct exchange of nutrients between the various layers of the skin: this leads in the long run to a further enlargement of the adipocytes, because the fat they contain cannot be easily utilised for energy purposes and tends to accumulate further, worsening the initial situation. The adipocytes, as they swell, compress the capillaries, which in turn pour plasma and toxins into the interstitial spaces, further clogging the local lymphatic and venous system: this is when the 'real disease', called cellulite, is generated, precisely when this vicious circle is established.

ii. Cellulite is not water retention

Water retention is the body's tendency to retain and accumulate fluid in the interstitial spaces, i.e. the spaces between cells. Due to the altered local circulation, not only liquids are retained but also toxins, further impairing the cell metabolism, which is already fatigued due to the poor oxygen supply caused by these conditions.

Water retention, therefore, is one of the causes of cellulite formation, as it clogs the local lymphatic system, causing inflammation of the subcutaneous connective tissue.

One should not mistake cause for effect, although the two are intrinsically connected.

73

iii.   Cellulite is almost never of only one type

Often several types of cellulite coexist in different areas of a person's body, e.g. type 2 cellulite on the thighs and type 1 cellulite on the arms. This is why we often speak of 'mixed cellulite', the most frequent form of which is a mix of water retention and adipose cellulite.

9. Conclusions

We have understood what cellulite is, how it manifests itself, what the main triggers are, but above all, we have learnt how difficult it is to manage as it is multifactorial in nature and presents itself in a way that is sometimes extremely different from person to person.

It highlighted the need for a multidisciplinary approach to defeat, or at least manage and limit, this pathology, which in many cases is not just a simple blemish, so much so that it conceals possible microcirculation problems, or inflammatory states that should not be overlooked.

We then analysed each of the triggers, showing possible solutions for each of them.

It is not possible to fight cellulite, if not through a holistic approach, which concerns our existence starting with our lifestyle, our clothing and footwear, our psycho-physical well-being, and ending with nutrition, supplementation and the most appropriate physical activity.

The analysis of the causes and possible solutions gives rise to the set of tips and suggestions presented in the various sections of the book to prevent the occurrence of this pathology: small changes to be included in our daily habits to live and feel better, allowing our organism to improve and limit, reduce or in some cases eliminate the problem. It is a bit like having a trunk with a treasure made up of many small gold coins: each coin has a value, but when added to the others it makes a real fortune!

Practical examples, summary tables, sample diagrams have been proposed, trying to use a language that makes these concepts accessible to all. Within the various sections, references have been included to expand on the concepts expressed and to consult the texts cited, where possible.

What is proposed is the fruit of the author's studies: it is a work of popularisation, and the reader is urged to seek advice from qualified medical, nutritional and sports personnel to solve the cellulite problem with an all-round approach.

The overview offered in this book is not meant to be exhaustive: it could never be. What is offered is an easy-to-read tool to better understand what we learn every day on the Internet, newspapers, magazines, TV, social and mass media in general. We are bombarded with information, often conflicting: it is really difficult to understand what has scientific merit, as opposed to what is an outright scam. In some cases, the difference is very subtle: this is the case of anti-cellulite diets that are valid for everyone, even promoted by 'eminent professionals'. Let us learn to always use our heads, with the benefit of the doubt: let us evaluate, document and turn to specialised and qualified personnel, certainly present in the place where we live, or in neighbouring areas.

There are no miraculous or pre-packaged recipes that are good for everyone: if only that were the case! Each case must be assessed on its own merits. However, having at least the minimum indispensable tools of knowledge becomes mandatory, so as not to fall into mistakes that can cause us health problems, or worse still, fall into the hands of unscrupulous charlatans.

To conclude, I want to leave in outline form a decalogue of tips for preventing, combating and overcoming cellulite at the table, already analysed in this book:

1. Drink the right amount of water

2. Favouring fibre-rich foods

3. Eat protein at least once a day

4. Do not overdo it with salt

5. Abolish or limit as much as possible alcohol, fried foods, coffee, cream, cold meats, chocolate, sweets, mayonnaise, packaged sauces, cooking stock cubes, tinned, oiled and canned foods

6. Simple cooking: steam, bake, in the oven, in non-stick pans, and season with raw olive oil

7. Fractionate calories: better to eat 5-6 small meals rather than 2 or 3 large meals

8. Supplementing the diet to improve metabolism, decongest and promote fluid reabsorption, tone capillaries and improve circulation

9. Check for food intolerances

10. Avoiding prolonged stress

Source: https://massimospattini.com/cellulite-i-10-comandamenti/

To this I would like to add another small reminder of 6 simple recommendations covered in the book:

1. Use suitable clothing, not too tight

2. Use suitable footwear, with not too high and comfortable heels

3. Avoid artificially sweetened drinks, alcohol, spirits and smoking

4. Taking time for oneself, to relax and if possible meditate, spending time outdoors whenever possible, adopting, as far as possible, a lifestyle that does not exceed the stress levels to be managed on a daily basis, working on oneself to banish negative thoughts and take on positive ones

5. Move, move and more move! Let's take long walks in nature...

6. Let us enjoy life intelligently, knowing that a degree of tolerance to all these recommendations is not only possible, but healthy (the infamous 80/20 Pareto Principle...)

We learn to set short-, medium- and long-term goals, to be verified through criteria that are as objective as possible. One objective at a time, to be achieved in a time frame we set ourselves, and then move on to the next one. The same method can be applied to introduce, for example, a new good habit every month (or every two months), so that after 4-8 weeks it has become a habit and not an imposition that, as such, would be set aside after a short time.

10.   Author's rights

Everything in this book is protected by copyright and intellectual property law.

It is strictly forbidden to copy, appropriate, redistribute or reproduce any phrase, content or image in this work without the express permission of the author.

Copying and reproduction of the contents and images in any form is prohibited.

Redistribution and publication of content and images not expressly authorised by the author is prohibited.

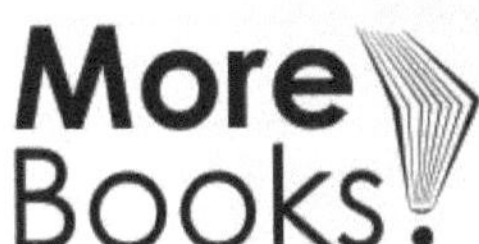

More
Books!

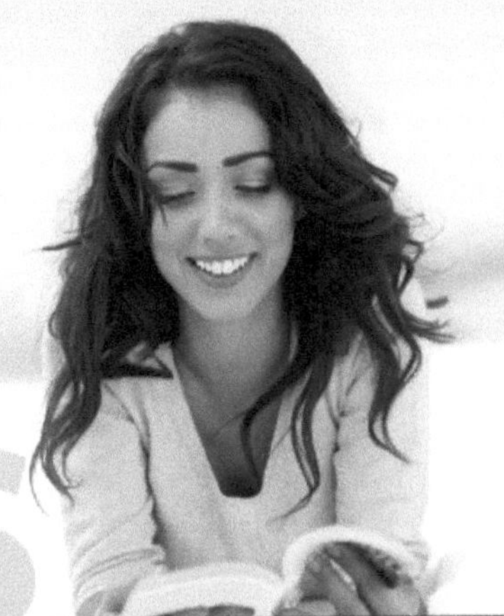

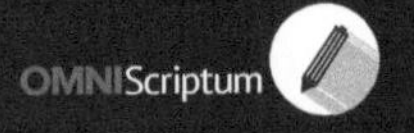

OMNIScriptum

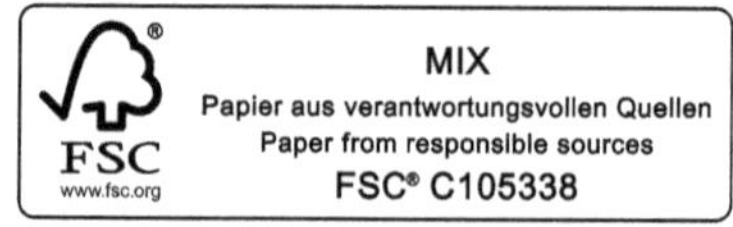

Printed by Books on Demand GmbH, Norderstedt / Germany